'Each person's experience of dementia is unique. This book, based on many years of first-hand experience, will help us all to find our own unique way to use creative approaches in caring. It will be an invaluable resource to support and inform our work.'

– Keith Walker, Executive Director, Befrienders Highland Ltd

'This book offers a different perspective in caring for those with dementia. Through a creative approach the author shows how it is possible to make connections and build relationships, with and without words. The process is described step-by-step, making it a valuable resource for anyone involved or interested in this field of work.'

– Julie Simmons, Adult Learning Strategy Officer, High Life Highland, Inverness

A CREATIVE TOOLKIT FOR COMMUNICATION IN DEMENTIA CARE

KARRIE MARSHALL

Jessica Kingsley *Publishers*
London and Philadelphia

Carl Sagan quote on p.84 reprinted with the permission of Little, Brown Book Group and Simon & Schuster, Inc. from *Contact* by Carl Sagan © 1985.

First published in 2016
by Jessica Kingsley Publishers
73 Collier Street
London N1 9BE, UK
and
400 Market Street, Suite 400
Philadelphia, PA 19106, USA

www.jkp.com

Library of Congress Cataloging in Publication Data
Marshall, Karrie, author.
 A creative toolkit for communication in dementia care / Karrie Marshall.
   p. ; cm.
 Includes bibliographical references and index.
 ISBN 978-1-84905-694-6 (alk. paper)
 I. Title.
 [DNLM: 1. Dementia--rehabilitation. 2. Communication. 3. Interpersonal Relations. WM 220]
 RC521
 616.8'3--dc23
                        2015027311

British Library Cataloguing in Publication Data
A CIP catalogue record for this book is available from the British Library

ISBN 978 1 84905 694 6
eISBN 978 1 78450 206 5

Printed and bound in Great Britain

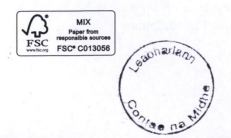

This book is dedicated to people who care for other people (for they are the students of love, mindfulness and creative communication), and to people diagnosed with dementia (for they are the teachers).

CONTENTS

INTRODUCTION

How do we best support a person's identity, relationships and emotional wellbeing through changes that occur as a result of brain disease, such as dementia?

Sometimes relatives and care staff reach a point where they are uncertain about how best to communicate or support someone; but with the support and tools shown here people find there are many ways. Communication is always possible.

This book contains tried and tested creative activities to support people to be themselves through a wide range of experiences. It is a toolkit for creative communication using step-by-step methods for interacting and making connections, with and without words.

For more than ten years the work was developed with people living with dementia; finding out what people prefer; learning what works best and why. The activities and approaches found here have received tremendously positive feedback.

As the disease progresses, the usual channels of communication can alter, leading to confusion, misunderstandings or upset. By using alternative means to exchange ideas or express feelings, people continue to have positive and meaningful interactions with each other.

Relationships may change as dementia progresses. This can be a difficult process for families and friends who rely on shared memories or clear roles and expectations of each other. Changes in recognition and communication also affect staff who build trust with the person they care for. But we can find new ways to be in relationships and spend quality time together without having to rely on words or memory. Every activity here can help with that process of adjustment.

Creativity helps to form a 'meeting space'. It adds a dimension to our engagement with each other that feels comfortable, and aids better communication. This becomes paramount when supporting someone who seems lost, anxious and confused.

Our brains are creative organs, constantly making neural connections, interpreting, processing and responding to stimuli. Different forms of dementia affect different parts of the brain, but we know from experience and from academic research that as people's brains change, creative aspects remain. It is through creative connections that we can support identities, relationships, self-expression, emotional wellbeing, independence and end-of life-care.

There are effective principles to learn along the way. Each chapter highlights a particular benefit that people living with dementia, family carers and staff identify as important. Tips, activities and approaches are shown to support benefits such as identity, memory, self-expression, relationships, emotional and spiritual wellbeing and peace. This promotes greater confidence in caring.

Attitudes towards living with dementia seem to be improving. There is wider acceptance that life can continue to be meaningful after diagnosis. We are more aware of the value of creative approaches to dementia care. There is greater focus on leading healthy lifestyles (for example, to reduce the risks of stroke that can cause vascular dementia) by reducing cholesterol, maintaining healthy weight, blood pressure and fitness, stopping smoking, reducing alcohol intake and exercising more.

It is important to be clear that dementia is not an inevitable outcome of older age. Most people do not get dementia, and people who do get diagnosed are not necessarily doomed to suffer. There are many ways to experience the disease. People can live well for several years, even through changes.

Whilst people speak about dementia as one thing, it is a collective term for different forms of brain disease causing a variety of symptoms, such as loss of concentration, confusion, loss of words, memory problems, deep suspicions, or changes in behaviour. Not every person experiences every symptom.

If the disease progresses, everyone involved must adapt to the conditions. This book describes ways to be supportive and continue through changes in abilities or understanding, using person-centred approaches. It shows that creative support is as important for the carer as for people diagnosed with dementia. There are parts of the book more applicable to family carers, but it is useful for all care staff to read and understand too.

Communication and interaction are extremely important. The lack of this has been picked up in many dementia care facilities. But we also know carers do the best with what they know. Sometimes all that stands in the way of communicating well is not having the confidence to try things differently.

The sense of loss (of words, memory, relationships, or familiarity) can feel overwhelming. Sometimes it seems as though the person with dementia can no longer communicate. But the real issue is that the usual channels of communication and topics of interest have changed, so we need to find new ways to connect.

Our own moods, beliefs and expectations have a significant impact on how we find others to be, so the book promotes self-awareness and self-care. Many of the activities are designed to soothe anxieties, release expression and share joyfully in the moment of 'now'. The importance of reducing stress for all involved cannot be overestimated.

Creative communication helps people discover that they do not have to rely on words or memory to spend quality time together. The author's work included analysing levels of engagement; noticing how alert or interested people were.

The activities were used with people diagnosed with a range of dementias (Lewy body; Alzheimer's; frontal temporal lobe; vascular dementia; Korsakoff's dementia; Binswanger's disease; dementia related to head injury or other illness) and with people at different stages of dementia, including people confined to bed, unable to lift their head from the pillow.

Observations were made about whether age or gender made a difference to the level of connection; how materials were used; how engaged carers were; the needs of people who also had different sight and hearing levels; interactions between people diagnosed with dementia and their carers; and identified benefits of activity were noted.

Whilst there are many strands to this, the overall conclusion is that creativity is all-inclusive. It bridges differences in language, culture, age and ability. Creativity is the means through which we engage and communicate. It is the golden thread that holds steady through the changes that disease may bring. There are myriad ways to be creative and all are valid. Important factors for effective communication include the following:

- Feel calm – calmness helps clarity, but it also helps the person with dementia feel more relaxed, which increases his or her ability to communicate.

- Open body language – be relaxed and friendly in your posture by using open gestures, smiles and eye contact.

- Listen with ears and eyes – be alert to non-verbal clues about how the person feels or what they mean.

- Calm voice – the tone of your voice can create a sense of safety. It can be bright and cheerful as well as calm. Invite people rather than demand.

- Respect personal space – be aware of how comfortable a person feels about physical closeness. This will be different on different days, depending on mood or pain levels, or context.

- Breathe – whilst we do all breathe, this is a reminder to be aware of your breath and the breath of the person you are communicating with. Slow your breathing to feel calm and relaxed. You can also connect through breathing together.

- Think creatively – be open to seeing things in different ways, and especially to noticing the skills, abilities and capacities that people living with dementia have.

Using this book

You will find the book is arranged in a series of benefits to enable you to turn to the chapters most relevant for your situation. Each chapter considers why a particular benefit is important, with references to support it.

However, if you read the book in sequential order you will find that I am describing journeys of self-discovery through dementia and caring that invite you to consider what dementia is teaching us.

SUPPORTING IDENTITY

Who am I?

This great philosophical question has fascinated humans for generations. How do I know who I am? When did I ever know who I was?

Does identity change, and if so, how do I recognise myself? In which part of me does my identity reside? Am I in all my body parts: limbs, organs, lymphatic and nervous systems? Or in my DNA, my blood-line and cells through history? We learn that our identity is in our unique finger swirls, ear shapes, eyes and dental patterns.

But there are other senses of identity concerning individuals and families living with dementia. We often think of identity in terms of the person's physical and relational place in society. Who are we in relation to others and the world? Where is our usual place? What is our regular role in our family or at work? We might say 'I am the sort of person who likes to…', which shows a sense of agency (control) over what we like to do, or say, or think, or feel, or remember.

It is this wider, more social sense of identity that people fear losing. In her online blog about living with younger onset dementia, Kate Swaffer (2015)[1] expresses a common fear:

> One major fear is the loss of self associated with dementia, and we face an existential crisis of identity. Our sense of self is shattered with this new label of dementia. Who am I, if I can no longer be a valued member of society? What if I don't know my family, if I don't know who I am and who I was? The inner fear of the loss of self, and loss of identity, is exacerbated by the outer stripping away of who we once were.

Kate's work beautifully describes fears and resolutions. She goes on to highlight the importance of family members, friends and carers supporting the person's identity by focusing on who they still are, and not on a bunch of symptoms labelled 'dementia'. This same message underpins the activities found here. There are many aspects to being human.

As awareness and understanding grow, our abilities to make meaningful connections deepen. The experience of working or living with people diagnosed with dementia usually requires us to adapt our own responses. It is good to know that we can continue communicating even beyond words and memory, as we learn to tune in to people we care for.

When we look at someone for the first time we often make a comparison with ourselves. We search for recognition and look for clues to relate to, things that feel familiar to us. 'Identity', from the Latin 'idem', means 'the same'. We are well practised at seeing what is like unto ourselves.

We are also attuned to spotting that which is different. It is a safety device and some people see difference more readily than others, but we all do it. Our response to changes in people living with dementia is important. The first few times a person says something that sounds unusual or strange can feel unsettling. If the exchange is unfamiliar, we may feel wary, which blocks the flow of communication. How we treat people in that moment can help or hinder their sense of identity.

The question 'Who am I?' has multiple answers. It is a mix of inner and outer factors influencing how we see ourselves and how others see us. Tom Kitwood (1997)[2] uses the term 'personhood' to express a range of factors that make up an individual. Life histories, sensory perceptions, environments, mental and physical health and the type of neurological impairment all affect how dementia is experienced.

We each have a distinctive life history. People growing up in the same family at the same time experience different opportunities and setbacks. There are differences in sensory awareness (eyesight, hearing, spatial awareness) that alter our experiences of the world in which we grow.

We encounter a variety of environments throughout our lives, depending on where we live, work or travel to. Our mental and physical health impacts on our quality of life, and shapes our abilities to cope with other diseases or long-term conditions. Various forms of dementia, combined with the degree to which someone has the disease, add to the mix that creates a unique experience.

Given all the variables, it is easy to understand why we should never make assumptions about someone else based on our own or anyone else's experience. Supporting identity is about delivering person-centred care. The focus is on the person, their ideas and preferences for the kind of life they want to live.

Cultural differences in valuing identity

Leichten, Wang and Pillemer (2003)[3] found there are cultural differences about the importance of individual identity. In independent countries we tend to place high value on autobiographical expression. Much of the work in dementia care aims to elicit personal memories to support individual identity. Autobiographical books and films are popular. Individuality, self-expression, uniqueness and autonomy are highly valued in Western Europe, the USA and Australia.

In East Asia, Africa, Southern Europe and Latin America there is greater focus on community harmony, social obligations and shared identity. In Asian cultures autobiographical accounts are rare and seen as undesirable (egotistical). 'I' is rarely found in Chinese poetry or prose (p.92). When asked by Leichten to recall childhood memories, respondents in a rural Indian community village seemed puzzled: 'They indicated that they thought the questions were irrelevant and that such memories were unimportant.'

It makes sense that in more rural areas communal memories are more important for survival. Remembering how to do things, or where water flows in summer, is more important than *'my first day at school'*.

In rural areas of the Scottish Highlands, too, it is clear to see that community history and shared memories are greatly valued. Whilst we may be placing emphasis on the person's ability to recall their personal history (and claiming that as evidence of their identity), we need to be mindful of the bigger picture. Some people's identities are extremely interlinked with their geography and history, more than with personal accounts of life events.

Identity and family carers

A diagnosis of a long-term condition like dementia affects the whole family. Many carers experience a sense of erosion, as though the disease of the person they support has consumed their own identity; and in care work, staff sometimes feel exhausted.

Caring for other people requires finding ways to feel resilient, which may involve asking for support. We do not support people who are ill by being ill ourselves. Doing meaningful and creative activities together can also help. It is important that carers (family or paid staff) try the activities for themselves. This will help maintain, or regain, a sense of purpose and enjoyment.

It is part of our role as carers, paid or unpaid, to be the most well versions of ourselves. This means supporting our own sense of identity. The activities are for everyone involved in the process of improving quality of life and supporting identity.

Activities to support identity

COLLAGE

Collage is an accessible form of artwork composed of materials such as paper, newsprint, photos, fabric, leaves, foil, tissue paper, etc. We use three different styles of collage:

- the first is a themed, paper-based collage that suits beginners as well as more established artists

- the second is a multi-media (and sometimes messier) form that usually requires a more solid base and stronger glue to hold objects in place

- the third style is designed for people who fear having a blank page. It involves gluing bits of paper onto a ready-made shape of something familiar (Chapter 6).

We use all three styles of collage with people living in all stages of dementia who require various levels of support. It is important to create our own collages alongside people. This gives clues about what is expected, and prevents us from taking ownership of their artwork.

COLLAGES ABOUT LIFE AND LIKES

The simplest version of this activity is to trust intuition to create the artwork. This works as well with people living with later stages of dementia, as it does with people in top jobs who want some fast therapeutic art!

The objective is not to think about the art or the outcome, but to notice what we are paying attention to. By choosing only the images, words or colours that catch our eye, we are doing the right thing regardless of the end result.

The materials include a piece of stiff paper (cartridge paper) to glue the images or decorative papers onto; a pile of magazines and wrapping papers for ripping; and a pot of glue with a glue brush. Scissors are not vital, but some people prefer them. A marker pen can be useful too. We tend to use aprons for this activity.

Set a timer for 15 to 20 minutes for pulling out images or patterns that seem to appeal most. If the person looks at an image for a second longer than other pictures, help them to rip it out! If a word or phrase catches the attention, tear it out! The images might be places, plants, furniture, cars, sunsets, clothes, animals… Pile up the images, patterns and phrases.

After the timer has sounded, spend a few minutes arranging the pile of gatherings on the paper. This is the point at which people start to register what they have been paying attention to. Glue everything in place. Study the work and see if the person wishes to add any words with a marker pen. (Note that people who do not speak can still often write or make a mark.)

The collages regularly show what people like or how they feel at this moment in time. Some themes are around colours and feelings more than tangible likes…but they are all interesting. One person created a collage using only two images. One image was a hand holding a diamond necklace. The other was a hand holding a flower. It was a striking piece of art.

Optional and very satisfying additions to this activity are to:

○   splatter the image with gold paint

○   glue a paper frame onto the work

○   photograph the image to create a card.

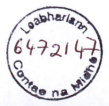

COLLAGE ABOUT ATTITUDES TO LIFE

This activity is done over a longer time period to include some discussion. The purpose of the activity is to create art about the attitudes we admire or wish we could develop in ourselves. The process means people can participate at different levels.

We each have personal and public identities. How we feel inside may not show to others, so sometimes the personal and public identities can seem far apart. People living with dementia may have that experience more acutely; if their words or memory are becoming confused, people around them begin making assumptions about the person's capacity. During this activity there have been people in their 90s who declared they have always wanted to be daring or wild!

We begin with a set of 'attitude' words written in bold letters on card. Often we try to find an image (an animal or an action shot) for each attitude as a back-up visual clue:

- playful
- determined
- glamorous
- wild
- lovable
- daring
- relaxed
- ferocious
- curious
- independent
- steady
- challenging
- focused

- ○ happy

- ○ adventurous.

Each artist (person with dementia, care staff, family carer) chooses an attitude that they *admire*, or that *they would most like to have*.

The materials are the same as in the first collage. Recreate the attitude word (or glue the chosen card) onto the page. Most people choose the centre, but there is no right or wrong way.

Again, set a timer for around 20 minutes for going through the magazines, ripping pages and tearing out images that seem linked to that attitude. What would a curious person be attracted to? What would surround a lovable person? What might a daring person get up to?

If you are unsure about whether the person understands the task, be confident about creating your own pile of images for your own collage. This helps the person see what the task is. We often find that people start ripping or pointing to images if we ourselves can remain calm and relaxed through the process.

Assemble the collection of images around the attitude word and glue them on. This task is not about things looking good or filling up the page. The activity is an arts project about attitudes to life, and in this respect we value every piece of work produced. If possible, spend time looking at each other's work and discuss personal attitudes to life.

CREATIVE BRAINS

The first version of this activity began as a drawing exercise. Whilst talking about the brain and neural networks, we drew some brain-shaped outlines on paper. People then created random lines across the space, representing their thoughts, and designed intersections for the pathways to link to. Some connections were plain square blocks, others were more flowery or intricate. This three- to ten-minute doodle exercise continues to be a lovely back-up activity.

MAKE A NEURON

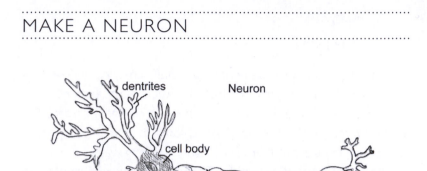

Figure 1.1: Diagram of a neuron

Our identities are inextricably linked to our unique sets of neural pathways and thought patterns. Sensory information received through our fingers, ears, nose, mouth, eyes and sensing abilities is interpreted by the brain, and a set of responses develops. Often, a range of factors at the time of the experience leads us to categorise the encounter as desirable or undesirable.

> In simple terms, if Amy is in her favourite place, with her best friends, when a song comes on the radio, her brain may create a neural pathway that always feels good around that song. No matter where Amy is, if her experience was intense enough (or if she frequently recalls the event), the neural pathway becomes reinforced, and she feels joy when she hears that song.

In contrast, if we find an experience highly embarrassing, or just plain boring, our brains create pathways that lead us to think in more negative terms every time we encounter a similar set of circumstances. Our regular responses become a part of who we are.

People say 'I always feel this when that happens.' It seems as though we have no control over the process, but with more awareness we can decide to think differently.

If you have ever tried to form a new habit you may know that establishing a new brain pattern can take several attempts… and possibly several years! So now is always a good time to begin forming new pathways. It can be useful to understand how the neural pathways work.

The next activity is popular with people of all abilities. It seems to help people understand why our brains need stimulation, and is useful for visualising new neural pathways. The activity involves making large-scale model neurons.

We have approximately 87 billion neurons or nerve cells carrying information to and from all parts of the brain. Some neurons are very long cells, stretching from the spinal cord through the arm to the fingertip, and from the spinal cord through the hip to the toe. Neurons connect with each other via signals passing across gaps between the neurons (synapses). There are some specialist neurons: for example, motor neurons specialise in signals to muscles for movement.

To make a neuron you will need several coloured fuzzy wires (approximately five or six per neuron) and a pair of scissors. Take a fuzzy wire and shape it into a ball…not too tight, just a loose ball shape. This represents the cell body. It is the centre of operations for the whole cell.

Pass another fuzzy wire through the ball to about half way along. Bend the wire and twist it, to form a twisted strand coming out of the ball. This part of the neuron is called the 'axon'. It is there to carry information away from the cell body towards another neuron.

The axon needs some protection and insulation. So take another fuzzy wire and fix it with a twist to the ball end of your axon. Now gently twist the new wire around the length of your axon, so that you can still see the axon through the gaps between the twists. This is creating the myelin sheath.

The myelin sheath is an insulator, which helps the electrical impulse of information to travel down the axon at high speed. Most people have some excess fuzzy wire at the end of their myelin sheath…you can make that into a bundle or a couple of branches at the end.

Return to the cell body ball and start creating tree-like structures called 'dendrites' by threading more fuzzy wires through the ball. We also cut pieces of wire to twist onto the longer pieces to create branches. These can be as long or as short as you desire. Once you have made your neuron you get to understand how it all works.

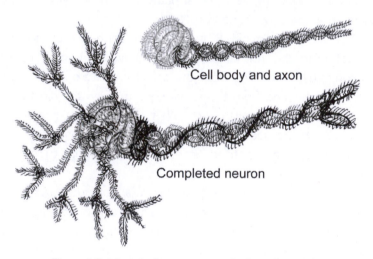

Figure 1.2: Model of a neuron made from fuzzy wires

The dendrites (tree-like branches) are there to capture information from nearby neurons to feed to the cell body. The cell body (ball) needs to build up an electrical charge to send information to the next neuron in the chain. So when it gets enough information through the dendrites, the electrical impulse shoots down the axon and out across the synapse to the dendrites on neighbouring neurons.

This is very exciting because the dendrites grow when we learn things. When exciting or interesting things stimulate us, our neurons respond. The opposite is also true. When we lack stimulation the dendrites shrink back into the cell body and the impulses cannot fire so well.

Make a few neurons and place them in a line with a gap between the end of one and the dendrites of the next. It is great to see a physical representation of a neural pathway. Some pathways will be well established. They will have been set up to fire in a particular way for many years to ensure that we move a certain way to clean our teeth, or drive the car, or think the same thoughts about particular situations.

If a neural pathway becomes blocked through damage or disease, the brain is naturally trying to form new pathways. Neuroplasticity (the brain's ability to reorganise itself) is an exciting area of study. Knowing that stimulation can help our dendrites grow gives people a boost.

CREATIVE BRAIN SCULPTURE

Another 'creative brains' activity can be done in two dimensions, or more effectively as a 3D sculpture. A few years ago, 55 people with dementia wanted to explore what was going on inside their brains. The topic was interesting but not very uplifting. We asked, 'What would you like to be going on inside your brain?' This raised the energy and created an array of beautiful and inspiring sculptures.

The first stage is to draw a large circle that represents a brain. The view is meant to be us looking down though the top of our head into our brain. Inside the circle, draw rough sketches of things you would like to be thinking about. Of the 55 sculptures created, no two were the same. They included soft furnishings, gardens, clouds, flowers, animals, homes, people, places, art, holidays, fishing, bread-making, music and walks.

The next stage is creating a shallow, bowl-shaped container for our preferred brain thoughts. We made the brain sculpture bases from chicken wire, shaped to resemble a neck with a bowl shape on top. This did involve a lot of wire cutting, so an effective alternative is to leave out the neck and create a large, papier-mâché bowl shape, using a bowl as a mould.

People probably need aprons and some like to wear thin gloves for this activity. If using a bowl as a mould, line it with greaseproof paper so that the papier-mâché object can be released away easily when dry. If you have a deep bowl, you can papier-mâché to about half the depth, so that people can see inside their finished sculptures.

There are different ways to work with papier-mâché, so do what feels familiar to you. One way is to tear newspaper into strips and 'paint' the strips them with a water-based glue to stick on the mould. It can be useful to use contrasting papers for each layer (e.g. newspaper followed by plain white paper), as then you can tell where you have been.

Do around six layers to create something sturdy enough to hold objects. Ideally, wait for the glue to dry in between each layer; otherwise the sculpture can take a couple of days to fully set.

While the sculpture is setting, the next task is to make or find things inspired by the initial sketches for inside the head. Use fabrics, netting, plastic ornaments and model flowers. Cut magazine images and stick them on card to create 3D effects. Sometimes people's creativity can take them far from their original sketch. This is perfectly allowable!

When the papier-mâché is dry and sturdy, paint it white. Once the paint has dried, the exciting phase begins. Fix the desirable thought objects inside the head sculpture. These sculptures make very interesting displays. They remind us all that we are all unique and intriguing.

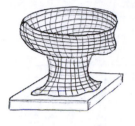

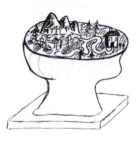

Figure 1.3: Brain sculpture

TREASURE CHEST

A treasure chest is a wonderful box of valuables. It is possible to buy blank treasure chests to decorate and fill, or you can use the image template (Figure 1.4) as a guide to create your own box. Use card of 300gsm thickness. The treasure chest measurements are approximately H 7 cm x W 9 cm x D 6 cm. Decorate the box with favourite wrapping paper. Even plain brown wrapping paper can look stunning with some gold glitter around the edges.

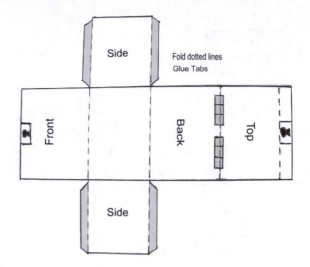

Figure 1.4: Treasure chest template: a) bottom of chest, and b) lid

Line the inside of the treasure chest with something that is meaningful to the individual. Some people prefer luxurious interiors such as soft fabrics, felt, velvet, or faux fur. Others like the idea of a pirate-style treasure chest. One man cut pieces of a map of his home area to line his box. Another used the colourful foil wrappers from sweets. One lady lined her box with old coins and notes from long-ago holidays in Greece and Italy.

We find that each person's treasure chest becomes an object worthy of sensitive and reverential treatment. They represent innermost valuables, even when apparently empty! One lady spoke about her box being full of love.

Most people like to place one or more physical representations of valuables. Recently, at a hospice, people chose sparkly jewels, wooden animals and natural objects such as pebbles and feathers. Treasure chests offer an opportunity to express identity. Each person can choose whether or not they wish to share what the treasure means to them.

....

LIFE-STORY BOOK
....

Life-story work has been used in social care work since the 1960s with children in care, and grew in the 1980s with adults living in long-stay institutions. Many care homes promote life-story work with people living in the care setting, involving their family members and staff.

Each story, whether it becomes a book or a performance, begins with some kind of narrative or memory. The following activity uses the book form that gives pleasure to so many people. I find most family members are keen to participate in life-story book making.

Before beginning the actual book, there are questions to consider for the person whose book it is:

○   What would it mean to me to do my life story?

○   Who would I like to show my story to?

○   Who would I not like to see my story?

○   Should I name other people in my life story?

○   What happens if I start remembering things that upset me?

○   What happens if I change my mind?

○   Where does my story work get stored?

○   Who owns my life story?

Some of these questions are ethical and need individual responses. In answer to the last question it is usual to assume that someone's life story belongs to that individual. This point can be argued if the person has not contributed to the making of their life-story book. A *biographical* account of someone's life is a culmination of other people's perceptions of him or her, and not the person's own views on how they lived their life.

Spend time exploring different themes. Ensure that the person living with dementia is involved right from the beginning. Use story-life focus topics such as those listed below to see which inspire most conversation. Do not push with questions. It is far better to write one or two topic headings in large writing on paper, and then offer the pen to the person. As with every activity, do your own version for yourself at the same time.

For example, begin with the topic of 'Family Life' in the middle of your page. Draw a line from the centre and add the word 'Dates'. Add your date of birth. Offer to support the person to add his or her own date of birth. Other dates may become apparent later, like date of acquiring driving license, or of marriage. Another line from the centre might be labelled 'Relatives'. List the most known relatives. Other lines could be places where we lived, family mealtimes, and family habits.

TOPICS FOR LIFE-STORY WORK:

- Family life
- School days
- Pets
- Occupations
- Interests
- Home and garden
- Holidays
- Spirituality
- Achievements
- Humorous moments
- Greatest adventure
- Wisdom gathered throughout life.

Use the topics to highlight positive aspects of life. These might be challenges that were overcome; proud achievements; important roles in life; and inspirational moments.

If the person has capacity to give consent, they need to understand what they are giving consent to. As a carer it is important to explain the purpose of the life-story work and go through the points above. Ensure that there are real opportunities for people to decide what they wish to include or leave out of their book.

WITHOUT CAPACITY TO GIVE CONSENT

If the person does not have capacity to give consent for recording their life stories, there may need to be discussion about the following:

- What purpose does a life-story book serve? Does it support other carers and staff to understand the individual, and so improve person-centred care? Does it give the person something to support their memory? Is there an argument against doing this work?

- Who will give consent to be recorded for the life-story work? Will a relative or guardian be willing to tell anecdotes or express appreciation for the person? Who has ownership of these stories…and of the final life-story book?

- How do we ensure that the life-story book is in a format that the person can access? Consider, for example, a DVD of images and people speaking; a book of stories and images to look at; a box of objects representing the person's life (see 'Memory Box' on page 53).

TIPS FOR WORKING WITH PEOPLE WHO DO NOT USE VERBAL LANGUAGE

Be curious about the person you are living or working with, and even if you have known them for years, consider the following questions. There is often a lot of information available about physical health or behaviours, because these are more easily recorded. The following questions help us consider the whole story:

Who is this person? What were they like as a child? What are their memories? What made them laugh? How did they cope with the tough times? Where have they ever felt safe or happy? Who were their favourite people? Whose voice or touch soothed them? Who read to them at night? What did they dream about? What funny incidents were they involved with? Where were their favourite places? What have they seen or heard? Who celebrated their milestones with them (first steps, or holding an object or signing)? What opportunities did they have to show their love? What inspired them to get up in the morning? Who did they turn to for support? What would they say they have lost in life? What would they say they have gained?

We may never know the answers, but it is important to keep acknowledging the vast life experiences and identities that people have. Stay open to the fact that each person has many stories, whether or not they can tell us. Look for clues, ask questions, listen with your ears and eyes. Most of all, value the whole person *and* their mysteries!

Life-story work is often labour-intensive, but the longer we give it, the more fruitful and rewarding the process becomes. People often want to tell their stories. It can take a few meetings for people to remember or say what really matters. Every life story is precious and intriguing. Treat each contribution with utmost respect.

DECORATED NARRATIVES

A narrative might be a moment in time, or a brief description of an aspect of life. The majority of my work uses narratives more than whole life stories. A sentence might be said by the person in passing, or by a relative. But it is significant. There is something expansive about moments in time that capture the imagination. A narrative can open the door to curiosity.

For example: one man's narrative was simply: 'I was a lighthouse keeper.'

Our curiosity asks: Where? How long for? What did you see? How did you feel? Did you get much sleep? What did you eat? Did you get lonely? What did you do? Were you ever afraid? Did you get stranded? Did you talk to the seagulls? Did you save lives?

Even without answers, a group of people who heard that narrative still had images of a lighthouse, sea, ships and gulls. Some went further and imagined mermaids, giant seahorses and treasure chests.

A piece of narrative can be decorated in ways that flow from the statement. Create a background of colour, images and words for the narrative to live in. These look wonderful when framed. You could use a deep-framed box to hold small objects related to the narrative.

Other short and poignant narratives we have worked with include:

'I worked in a beautiful gown shop.'

'I had six children and made all their clothes.'

'I worked on the railway. I checked the lines.'

WORD PORTRAITS

This is a short activity that can be used in a variety of ways, and it suits people who can write or speak. Each person is given a drawing of a basic body template and asked to write their own name on it. The main question they are to answer is 'Who am I?'

Each person lists around the body any words that describe who they are. This can be done for example, around nationality, life roles, physical features, health and interests.

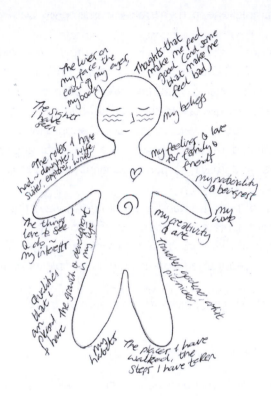

The lines on my face, the colour of my eyes, my body

Thoughts that make me feel good (and some that make me feel bad)

The sights I have seen

My beliefs

The roles I have had ~ daughter, wife, sister, mother, writer

My feelings & love for family & friends

My nationality & belief

The things I love to see & do ~ my interests

My creativity & art

Travelling, gardening, art picnics!

Challenges that I am & the growth & development I have

My values

The places I have walked, the steps I have taken

Figure 1.5: Word portrait

When people share their results, other thoughts are triggered about how we each define ourselves and who we identify with. Sometimes people (including relatives and staff) are surprised by what they listed first on the templates.

PUPPETS

Puppets made in our likeness can be extremely powerful and effective for self-expression. Puppetry communicates well because it connects on an emotional and often non-verbal level. There is humour and vulnerability combined with visual and moving impact.

A simple activity involving model theatre puppetry is to create photo-head–cartoon-body puppets. You will need copies of photographs of peoples' heads and shoulders approximately 2–4cm square (so the individual can see their head), and glued onto a piece of card. Next support the person to choose an ideal body or clothing from a magazine to glue onto the card below the head.

Have a selection of individual identities for different moods or life phases. These are often extremely funny, but also very expressive of who we are, were, or would like to be. One man wanted his head placed on the body of a mountain climber, as he had enjoyed walking in the hills of Scotland. A lady put her head onto the body of a tennis champion, as she had always loved tennis but never found the time to play.

Identity is greater than a diagnosis

Create opportunities to play around with the concept of our many selves. People become limited by labels or roles assigned by others. Our identities are greater than a diagnosis, or the role of a patient or carer. Feil (1993)[4] urges us to look beyond the disease and symptoms to the person. She writes about people with dementia as having 'a human knowing' and 'humanity that shines through'.

When people fail to recognise the existence of that humanity and knowing, they reduce their expectations of people with dementia. Our expectations cause us to see what we expect to see. Expectations create the range of what we believe others are capable of, and delineate the opportunities made available. The ideal habit would be to practice greater expectation without putting pressure on anyone to 'perform'.

Sometimes carers question whether a person in later stages of dementia is aware of their identity. Sabat and Harré (1992)[5] believe we have personal and public identities. They state that individual public personae, or our outer 'selves', can be damaged by people's failure to understand the person, but the personal identity still remains intact. When given the right opportunity, which is usually a creative, safe and enjoyable environment, people who may not have spoken or engaged for months, or even years, reveal who they are.

Lesser A.H. 2006[6] philosophically considered whether a person with 'serious dementia' retains their identity. He suggested that identity is not destroyed, nor should relationships end and the past should not be invalidated. Thus, Lesser concluded that a person does retain their identity. Many family carers who witness changes may argue this point...but it is worth taking into account. What supports identity? We support identity by accepting people in any given moment. If we practise this for ourselves, we will be very good at doing this for others.

References

1. Swaffer, K. (2015) 'Identity, isolation and dementia.' Available at http://kateswaffer.com/2012/08/07/identity-isolation-and-dementia. Accessed on 2 July 2015.
2. Kitwood, T. (1997) *Dementia Reconsidered: The Person Comes First.* Buckingham: Open University Press.
3. Leichten, M., Wang, Q. and Pillemer, D.B. (2003) 'Cultural Variations in Inter-dependence and Autobiographical Memory: Lessons from Korea, China, India, and the United States.' In R. Fivush and C.A. Haden (eds) *Autobiographical Memory and Construction of a Narrative Self: Developmental and Cultural Perspectives.* London and Hillsdale, NJ: Lawrence Erlbaum Associates.
4. Feil, N. (1993) *The Validation Breakthrough: Simple Techniques for Communicating with People with Alzheimer's-type Dementia.* Baltimore, MD: Health Professions Press.
5. Sabat, S. and Harré, R. (1992) 'The construction and deconstruction of self in Alzheimer's disease.' *Ageing and Society 12*, 443–461.
6. Lesser, A.H. (2006) 'Dementia and Personal Identity.' In J.C. Hughes, S.J. Louw and S.R. Sabat (eds), *Dementia: Mind, Meaning, and the Person.* Oxford: Oxford University Press.

∘ 2 ∘

SUPPORTING MEMORY

The brain stores memories in different spaces, through processes that make connections between neurons carrying different pieces of information. Neurons are the nerve cells that connect with each other. The neural pathways pass information around the brain and body. We might associate a smell with a memory of a feeling, or an image with a memory of a sound, through the neural connections. However, brain disease, brain damage and stress affect the way memories are stored and retrieved.

The thought of being without memory concerns people. There is a belief that memory makes us 'more real' and validates our past. Relatives fear being forgotten. Individuals fear losing the ability to remember where or who they are. But there are different forms of memory, being stored in different places. Some are about factual knowledge; others about personal experiences.

There are memories about the meaning of words; or what objects look like and how they move. Some memories have been reinforced over decades, whilst others are more transient. We have conscious memories that we try to recall, and memories that live in subconscious space and enable us to do things without much effort. Not all of these memories are affected at the same time or to the same degree.

Harrison *et al.* (2007)[1] refers to a 'preserved implicit memory' system in people living with dementia, where previous experience or familiarity of something enhances the person's ability to function in a similar situation, or to recall how to do something (procedural memory). Activities towards a daily life task or a creative activity do not need the words. They may include such activities as cutting paper, sewing, knitting, digging, peeling, polishing, brushing, sandpapering and dancing. We have done all of these tasks with people in late stages of dementia who had word loss or confusion, but who still had procedural memory.

When we encounter anything, there is an array of information that arrives via different senses to associated parts of the brain. For example, if we go to the park, our brains receive data about the sight of sunlight on the fishpond; the dogs chasing after a stick; the people pushing prams or riding bicycles. Information includes images of the faces we see; the sounds of the birds, barks and laughter. We might register information about the smells; the flowers and grass; the sensation of the weather and temperature on our skin; the words we speak or hear someone else speak; and how we feel about being there. All these separate pieces of information are received in different parts of the brain.

Sensory memories appear initially to be stored in the outer layer (cortex) of the brain, and are then gathered in spaces around the hippocampus deeper in the temporal lobe. The memories are connected together, so, for example, the experience of the park becomes one memory and not a series of bits of information. The hippocampus does much of this processing and organises where the memory will be stored and how it can be retrieved. It is involved in storing long-term memories and in moving some of them into even more permanent storage areas.

If memories are repeated enough times, the connections become strong enough to be independent of the hippocampus. The retrieval is direct and can be triggered by any of the pieces of information awakened. Hearing the word 'park'; seeing sunlight on water; hearing a dog bark…any one of these could be the point of entry to the whole memory. The person living with dementia may not be able to say what they are thinking, but the brain is constantly working.

In Alzheimer's disease there can be issues around taking in new information. This may be due to damage in the hippocampus area where cells usually process new information. Without the processing part, information remains unconnected. The experiences are stored as that sound, this fact; that face, this place, that sentence, this feeling. This is harder to make sense of and difficult to express or recall.

Without a means to remember the whole experience, the memory seems lost. This explains how long-term memories can be intact, whilst recent information is not recalled. People living with short-term memory loss can still enjoy life-story work and reminiscence activities. They may need more practical support to remain independent.

Emotional elements are often still intact, even when the person cannot recall the facts of a memory. Emotions are processed in a deeper part of the brain (the amygdala), which is affected much later than the hippocampus, and sometimes is not affected at all. This is why emotional connection with people is so important. People may not recall your interactions, but they recognise how the encounter felt.

Frontal temporal lobe dementia (FTD) affects different memory functions. The disease may be in parts of the brain that affect behaviour (called behavioural variant FTD) or language comprehension and speech (called progressive aphasia). Language difficulties occur when the person has problems remembering what words mean. This semantic knowledge is vital for us to understand meaning and to see how words relate to each other.

Martin and Chao (2001)[2] identified part of the left frontal lobe as important for semantic memories, and the temporal lobe for memories specifically about the naming of objects.

If object-naming knowledge cannot be recalled, it is difficult for people to find the right word or to understand the meaning of other people's words. This does not in any way mean the person is unintelligent. Their brains are working extremely hard to reconnect to find the missing information.

Allow time and use visual aids for conversations. Anxiety and stress about the loss of words can increase language difficulties. Any pressure to converse can increase the hormone cortisol, which is released under stress. Lupien *et al.* (2005)[3] showed that high levels of cortisol intensify problems with memory and cognitive performance. Be gentle, and use images or physical and creative activities to support people with frontal temporal lobe dementia.

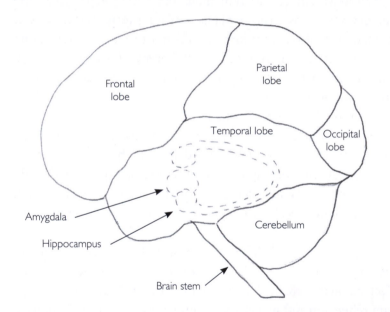

Figure 2.1: The lobes of the brain

Many years of experience in dementia care show us that people can still live meaningful and enjoyable lives with different forms of memory loss. The experience is very individual because it is influenced by personal attitudes to life, other people's responses and the nature of the brain disease.

Some people are aware of difficulties in recalling details about subjects they used to feel passionate about. This awareness of the loss of memory can be very painful. Strategies can be developed, such as the gathering of relevant information or photographs, to help the person recall their own experiences. But more important than any of that is the ability of the carer to help the individual feel at ease, even in the worst of times.

In some situations carers discover relief in acknowledging the loss of memory with the person they support. This kind of discussion requires empathy and trust in the process for moving through the problem to a place of acceptance. But not everyone wants to have that conversation. Some people develop tactics to cover up their memory loss. These include joking around the subject, or using practised sentences to throw people off the topic. Examples may include:

'That was in the past; you're a bit behind the times aren't you!'

'Why are you asking me about that? Get your own hobbies to talk about!'

An insightful carer can usually tell when a person is struggling with memory loss, and go with the flow of the conversation. Memory recall can be elusive. Our role is always to find the human connection that feels most comfortable and relaxing. If the subject is causing the person to feel inadequate, upset or frustrated, it is vital to change the interaction. There is nothing to be gained from insisting a person remembers something they simply cannot at this moment in time.

Individual and social memory

Assmann (2008)[4] described memory in relation to identity and time. This is shown on three levels: individual memory, spanning the person's life; social or communicative memory, spanning three or four generations; and cultural memory that may encompass over 3,000 years and more into mythical times. Here we can see how each level might be of use in dementia care:

Our *individual memory* has varying years of usefulness, depending on how memory is stored and recalled, and whether or not it is affected by brain disease. Typically this is the type of memory (autobiographical memory) that most people in western culture focus on in dementia care. Memory books and photo albums, home videos and memory quilts all support a person's explicit memory, to consciously remember who they are.

The *social or communicative* timeframes move with the generations, typically spanning three or four generations over a period of 80 to 100 years. This type of memory recall works well in groups (family or community) that include people living with and people living without dementia. Families or friends may recall more general events. These could be life events such as births and marriages, but could also be recipes or the family ornaments.

There is a collective retelling of social stories that can trigger spontaneous autobiographical expression. We find this happens, for example, during community history projects, as well as after singing community songs together. A relevant long-term memory may be triggered. Someone who cannot recall who their partner is may still be a fount of knowledge on local history.

It is also worth considering what opportunities exist for people to tell their stories. As children and growing adults, we encounter several social occasions in which we can tell and retell our personal or social memories. If people become isolated through illness or disability, there are fewer chances to recount memories, or strengthen those neural pathways.

The third level of memory in relation to identity and time is *cultural memory*. This forms the background to everything else we experience in society. Cultural memory has advantages and disadvantages. A shared history focused on people's ingenuity and ability to adapt will promote a healthier nation than one that is focused on war and conflict. Cultural attitudes may be so old that they are difficult to shift. We each grow up in pervasive cultures, unaware of their influence until we encounter a different culture.

We unconsciously develop ways of doing things, based on what those around us do. The way we greet someone is a good example of this. People with dementia may well recognise culturally important gestures. Cultural objects are also important for memory. Tourist shops sell souvenirs because people want physical mementos of the place. Souvenirs can inspire conversations and trigger memories of national or social events.

Cultural memories encourage people to remember selective aspects of history and 'ignore' the parts that are less tolerable (e.g. slavery or other crimes against humanity). In a BBC programme about collective memory, Bourke (2013)[5] talked about the silence people know they must keep for a few generations when memories are too painful and not conducive to creating a better world.

Carers need to be sensitive to individuals' need to 'remember' or 'forget'. Understanding relevant collective memory is helpful for supporting people more mindfully. Cultural memory is also found in rituals, festivals and celebrations around the world:

- Burn's Night in Scotland is over 200 years old.

- Thanksgiving Day in America is over 400 years old.

- Aoi Matsuiri in Kyoto, Japan, is approximately 1,400 years old.

- Hari Raya (or Eid al-fitr) that ends the Muslim Ramadan is also approximately 1,400 years old.

- Christmas Day has been celebrated in the UK for over 1,600 years.

- Diwali (festival of lights) in India is over 2,000 years old.

- The Chinese New Year festival is over 3,000 years old.

These festivals and arts (including architecture, statues, songs, poetry and text) carry cultural information that can support memory in a much wider context. Famous paintings of historical subject matter include 'The Death of Nelson' by American artist Benjamin West (1805); 'Guernica' by Spanish artist Pablo Picasso (1937); 'Rain, Steam and Speed (The Great Western Railway)' by English painter Joseph M. W. Turner (1844); and 'Sic Transit Gloria Mundi – Retreat From Moscow' by Richard Caton Woodville (1911). Each art piece depicts a moment in history captured in brushstrokes.

Since the 1870s a form of American history has existed through the poetry of Henry Wadsworth Longfellow. Shakespeare's plays offer artistic versions of English history and medieval society. Whether or not the works are remembered, they can be inspiring points of connection. When we hear ancient Greek classics such as the *Iliad* or the *Odyssey* by Homer, we become part of a long line of people who have shared that experience for well over 2,000 years.

This concept of continuing history and memory long after an artist or writer has died is important in dementia care. Individual memory may disappear but we continue to be connected through community and collective memory. People understand the value of recording personal or cultural history, not so much for themselves, but for family members and the people who are yet to come.

Explicit memories

Chen and Conway (2008)[6] explain that memory involves many different forms of knowledge in a wide range of contexts. 'Explicit memory' is the term used with reference to our memory about what we know. They refer to Tulving (1972)[7], who first proposed two different forms of long-term memory: the *semantic* (factual knowing) and the *episodic* (more personal remembering).

Someone may recall facts such as the name of a songwriter or the year of recording. This is an example of explicit memory, as it is about factual information. We usually refer to this as 'general knowledge'. Quiz puzzles and board games with set questions and answers can be fun for people who enjoy these factual pieces of information.

Others like to focus on memories linked to the senses and emotions. These are more personal or episodic memories. For example, a person may recall feelings about owning a record, or describe where he or she was when it was played. These memories may be hidden for a while, but they are classed as explicit or conscious memories. All forms of life-story work described in the preceding section on 'individual and social memory', and the use of images and physical ornaments, help support this episodic memory.

Implicit memories

Implicit memories (sometimes called procedural memories) refer to 'knowing how to do things'. As mentioned above, this can be in the subconscious memory. Physical activities support people to feel more useful and can stimulate these memories. We have noticed that repeating movements seems to improve the person's ability to recall the movements more quickly each time, even whilst other memories may be in decline. Dance routines; chair exercise; drama; or more practical activities are valuable ways to connect.

Activities to support memory

Whilst the following activities are used to support memory, their primary aim is to build a stress-free, enjoyable and easy connection. Within this environment, the person stands a much greater chance of recalling memory. Families have described some of these activities as therapy for carers. There is a sense of being able to do something positive in the face of the disease.

ENLARGED PHOTO ALBUM

When living with dementia, people need all the clues they can get. Create an album that consists of enlarged family photographs to give every opportunity for the person to see them clearly. Create large-print labels with the person. Decorate the pages. Use copies of photos in case the originals become soiled. Make the sharing of the album a regular and joyful event.

Never use the album as a means to 'test' the person on their memory. It is saddening to watch someone with dementia disengage from the photo album. This tends to occur when family members or care staff repeatedly ask, 'Who is that?' or 'Do you remember that day?' They could instead be using the photo album as a source of loving connection and stories. They could even just sit together in relaxed silence sharing a book of faces and places – no pressure required.

MUSIC OF THE ERAS

If you know a person's life story, or even the era and geography of his or her younger years, it is possible to gather songs and music from that time and place. Play extracts of music and notice which ones resonate most. Compile a list of music for different moods, and if possible create CDs or iPod playlists for the person to use as and when desired.

You may get a sense of the type of music that would have been popular when an individual was a young person. Try and discover the music they first bought or danced to. Music accompanies so many rites of passage. Just think of how popular BBC Radio 4's *Desert Island Discs* programme is, where people associate pieces of music with meaningful life experiences.

People become more alert, smile or exchange a look when they hear a personal favourite. The brain is more stimulated and people may speak more or engage with other activities. It is possible to hear a wide range of music and songs on the Internet (on YouTube, Spotify and iTunes). This makes it easier to try out a few tracks and notice what the person prefers. Music and lyrics are emotive, so tears and laughter are common. It is great to be able to share these experiences.

You can buy individual tracks and put them onto a CD or an MP3 player. With comfortable headphones the person can listen to their favourite tracks. If you leave the person alone, ensure that they can remove their own headphones, or check after 15 minutes.

If you are not sure what song would suit the person, sing chorus parts until you find one that resonates. Singing together can be inspiring. People find themselves smiling and nodding at each other. Such activities promote equality.

There is online support for creating personal playlists.

MY MOTHER'S BATHROOM

Fragrances have an evocative capacity that transports us via memories to people, places, activities and emotions we have experienced. The smell of baby powder has been popular in the UK since the 1940s. During discussions about favourite smells through the decades, participants listed Lux and Pears soap. Other favourites included roses and lavender.

Perfumes were often reserved for special occasions and bought as gifts. *Chanel No. 5* (launched in the 1920s) was a hoped-for gift. In the 1950s and 60s the sweet-smelling woodland flower *Lily of the Valley* by Yardley was popular. Other items in the bathroom may include Morny's *French Fern* bath cubes and talcum powder.

Men's aftershave from the 1950s included *Floris No. 89* and *Old Spice*, which reminds people of Christmas. The Wrights Coal Tar strong-smelling antibacterial soap was first created in 1860 and is still used (tea-tree oil has now replaced coal tar). Other reminiscent bathroom smells included disinfectant and pine.

The activity can start with looking at images of the items and then describing or sketching the bathroom that people remember, or a bathroom they would like to have. It is also possible to buy some of the fragrances and use them to stimulate memories. Many people enjoy the aromas, and this is an activity that can be done a few times.

Alternatives to the bathroom theme would be to include general household smells such as window cleaner, bread, engine oil, paraffin heaters, cut grass, etc.

HIGH DAYS AND HOLIDAYS

Can you imagine the thrill and excitement of leaving behind all the usual routines to go somewhere else for a change of scenery? Where would you go? A lot of enthusiasm is in the planning, raising the anticipation of having a lovely time.

The joy of this activity is in the planning. You do not physically have to go anywhere. Alternatively, you may like to hold an event for an hour or so to make it special. The purpose is to create a sense of wonderment together.

This activity could begin by listing and discussing all the high days and holidays common to the person's culture. In the UK this could include:

- birthdays
- Valentine's Day
- Christmas
- Easter
- Bonfire Night
- family events
- royal events.

Some people talk about regular weekly dances they used to attend, or events like the circus coming to town, and trips to a holiday beach, pleasure gardens, stately homes. Some recall riding on a steam train or visiting the zoo, having a picnic, being at the fairground, on a boat, or at their favourite aunt's house. All of these ideas are inspiration for planning a special day, creating an itinerary of what to see and how to get there – or offer ideas to recreate some of the magic at home.

For other ideas look up national and international celebration or commemoration days for people to mark at home, such as World Mental Health Day (10 October); World Poetry Day (21 March), Earth Day (22 April), International 'Talk Like a Pirate' Day (19 September).

PARLOUR GAMES

Indoor games became popular in the late 1800s in Victorian Britain and America. You do not need a parlour (extra livingroom) to play these games. The main materials required are paper, pens and dice. The amusement stimulates different neural pathways. Such games include:

1. 'Consequences' – imagination, language, dexterity
2. 'Beetle' – dexterity, maths
3. 'Fish on the Dish' – physical (oxygen), problem solving
4. 'Pin the Tail on the Donkey' – balance, listening
5. 'Charades' – imagination, language, memory.

An additional outcome from playing these games is the stimulation of memory about family gatherings or birthdays.

HOW TO PLAY 'CONSEQUENCES'

The game is traditionally played by writing single words or short phrases in answer to a set of standard questions, to create a mini story. The players begin all at the same time, by answering the first question and folding the paper to hide what they have written, before passing it to the next player. The next player each writes their answer to the second question, then folds the paper and passes it on to the next player. This continues until all the questions are answered.

1. Once upon a time there was a man – what sort of man?
2. What was his name?
3. And there was a lady – what sort of lady?
4. What was her name?
5. Where did they meet?
6. What was the man wearing?
7. What was the lady wearing?
8. What did he say to her?
9. What did she say to him?
10. What was the consequence? (What happened?)

'Consequences' can also be played in a drawing version, where the first player draws the head, passes it unseen (by means of folding) to the second player, who draws the body, and passes it on to the third player, who draws the legs. Unfolding the paper then reveals the composite person or creature.

'THE MINISTER'S CAT'

All players sit in a circle. The first player describes the minister's cat with an adjective beginning with the letter 'A' (for example, 'The minister's cat is an adorable cat'). Each player then does the same, using different adjectives starting with the same letter. Once everyone has done so, the first player describes the cat with an adjective beginning with the letter 'B'. This continues for each letter of the alphabet.

In an alternative version, the first player describes the minister's cat with an adjective beginning with the letter 'A', the second with the letter 'B' and so forth, going around the circle.

In both variants, a player is 'out' of the game if they are unable to think of an adjective, or if they repeat one already used. Players may clap in unison or speak in a rhythmic manner during the game, setting the pace for each player to speak his line; if a player falls too far behind the pace while thinking of an adjective, he or she may also be declared 'out'.

MEMORY BOX

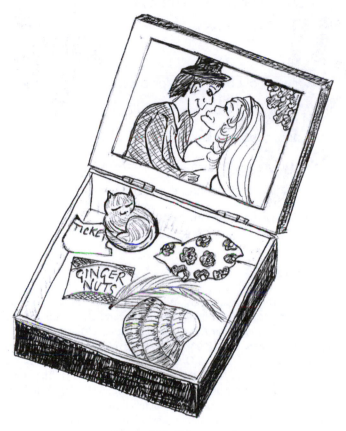

Figure 2.2: A memory box

Memories can be stored in places within and without us. The following ativity creates a more hands on memory aid than a photo album. The memory box contains objects that represent memories or experiences. If no history is known and the person is in later stages of dementia, the activity can be more about commemorating current times.

Decorate a shoebox with favourite paper or material. (Shoe shops usually have spare boxes to give away.) Consider questions from the life-story book activity (Chapter 1) and gather objects, photos and materials that represent the person's life events. Another option is to gather what people currently like and experience:

○ labels off favourite foods

○ poems

○ photocopies of book jackets or covers

○ the Christmas joke that made him or her smile

○ small ornaments of pets

○ pieces of fabrics the person likes, sewn together

○ driftwood, feathers, cones, etc., from walks

○ postcards or tickets from places visited.

References

1. Harrison, B.E., Arbor, A., Kim, J. and Whall, A.L. (2007) 'Preserved implicit memory in dementia: A potential model for care.' *American Journal of Alzheimer's Disease and Other Dementias 22*, 4, 286–293.
2. Martin, A. and Chao, L.L. (2001) 'Semantic Memory and the Brain: Structure and Processes.' *Current Opinion in Neurobiology 11*, 2, 194201.
3. Lupien, S.J., Schwarts, G., Ng, Y.K., Fiocco, A. *et al.* (2005) 'The Douglas Hospital longitudinal study of normal and pathological aging: Summary of findings.' *Journal of Psychiatry and Neuroscience 30*, 5, 328–334.
4. Assmann, J. (2008) 'Communicative and Cultural Memory.' In Erll, A. and Nünning, A. (eds) *Cultural Memory Studies: An International and Interdisciplinary Handbook.* Berlin / New York: de Gruyter.
5. Bourke, J. (2013) Interview in 'The Why Factor' on BBC World Service Radio. Available at www.bbc.co.uk/programmes/p014knyn. Accessed on 6 July 2015.
6. Chen, G. and Conway, M.A. (2008) *Memory in the Real World.* New York: Psychology Press.
7. Tulving, E. (1972) 'Episodic and Semantic Memory.' in E. Tulving and W. Donaldson (eds) *Organisation of Memory.* New York/London: Academic Press.

∘ 3 ∘

SUPPORTING RELATIONSHIPS

We are who we are in relation to ourselves, others and the universe. We are constantly in relationship with *something* or *someone*. And yet many people diagnosed with dementia experience isolation, exclusion and loneliness. Why does that happen? What is required to change it?

When someone is diagnosed with dementia there is usually a change of perception by the person about him or herself, and by family relatives and/or care staff. The person is now seen through a filter called 'dementia' that highlights differences. It notices forgetfulness. It alerts people to strange sounding sentences. The filter registers every time the person misplaces an object or forgets to do something. To be seen through such a filter is an alienating experience.

The person living with dementia (particularly in the early stages) is almost living under a different set of rules to those who are not diagnosed. People who live without dementia are allowed to forget names or misplace things without that being noted or remarked upon. They are permitted to get confused about what they are doing next, or what day it is, or to miss an appointment, because the incidences are occasional and recoverable.

Of course, people diagnosed with dementia may be showing more symptoms and on a more regular basis. The prompts and clues are not enough when the brain is damaged, so people need more support. But this must be inclusive and empowering, focused on capacity, not on decline. When the focus is on incapacity, the perspective of the person leads to unnecessary discrimination. This is something we can address.

Crocker and Garcia (2009)[1] refer to the threat posed to the targets of stigma, regarding the self-image they want others to validate and acknowledge. If having dementia is regarded as inferior to not having dementia, it is easy to see how people with dementia feel devalued. Negative media images further reinforce this possibility. Crocker and Garcia use the phrase 'downward spiral' for this kind of experience, but they believe it is possible to create upward spirals through open and constructive communication.

> If all victims wait for perpetrators to change their behaviour, the downward spiral will continue unabated. The best possibility for creating change is starting with the self…where one has leverage to create upward spirals in intergroup relations.
>
> (Crocker and Garcia 2009)

This may involve the person with dementia expressing feelings of vulnerability in this situation, or being fearful of being devalued in this interaction. Speaking the truth in this way enables other people to be more aware of how they are responding, and to create a more equal and co-operative connection.

You may have had the experience of meeting someone who you notice has great social skills, is friendly and feels easy to be with, when suddenly you notice a difference. Perhaps the person declares a belief in direct contrast to yours, or speaks unfavourably about someone you like. There's a moment when the difference causes you to be more wary and to hold back a little.

This response of distancing oneself can also happen in interaction with someone living with a disease that affects their language or conduct. For example, one very affable man was able to hold social conversations and entertain others with jokes, but his mood could change instantly into one of suspicion and coldness. For new people this behaviour was utterly confusing and their withdrawal was palpable, which the man was keenly sensitive to. This would exacerbate the situation, leading him to feel more suspicious. However, those who knew the man were able to divert his attention to a familiar or uplifting topic, which helped him pick up his jovial manner again.

When someone behaves differently, such as becoming confused, or makes a delayed response to something that was said a few sentences before, or does not engage in an expected manner, there is a tendency to respond in ways that are exclusionary.

By raising awareness of our own responses, we can become better at helping those around us to support people living with dementia. Family members notice the difference it makes when they are more confident about dealing with issues such as their partner or parent saying something rude in public. If they can find the place of humour, or the path of diversion, people around them seem more able to cope, rather than reject the person with dementia. The opposite of that is also true.

If a carer feels excruciatingly embarrassed by the behaviour or comments of their relative, people around them may mirror their awkwardness and resistance to the situation. The consequence of these responses is isolation of the person with dementia. Some families stop going out because of the fear of embarrassing social situations, thus leading to more isolation.

Awareness of the issues faced by people living with dementia is growing, and this can help families, friends and care staff be more understanding and less afraid. The value of being in a loving relationship cannot be overestimated, but it not always easy.

Family difficulties

Often one member of the family becomes the main carer. This may not be a conscious decision, but a default position (husband or wife) or as a result, for example, of a son or daughter's geographical or occupational situation. Sometimes the family carer can feel unsupported or isolated. A person with dementia may appear 'fine' every time relatives visit; the fresh energy or novelty of a visit may well stimulate the person with dementia so that all appears well to the visitor. Lack of insight and understanding into the 24-hour caring situation can cause many problems. The carer himself may feel he is not competent, particularly when the person with dementia seems to engage readily with visitors, or recognises a visitor and not the carer.

These effects, painful or calculated as they may seem, are really just indications of how energy is flowing in and around the brain. We are all attracted to fresh, bright, uplifting energy. We naturally seek new experiences for interest and curiosity. It is why creative activities are so important, not just for the person with dementia, but for the carers to experience joyfulness too.

Carers notice a difference when they remove themselves from a difficult situation and return with a higher and more positive energy. But to find that fresh energy requires time for self-nurturing. Some family carers have spoken about the importance of having a garden shed or a small summerhouse that is private and peaceful – a space to visit, even for ten minutes, to recharge. Put a garden chair outside the backdoor just for you!

If carers become defensive, angry, frustrated, guilty or jealous, what they need is a good deal of tea, kindness and empathy. People need to know they are appreciated and loved. It is really good when they are reminded that they are actually doing very well. Sometimes all of that support has to come from within the carers themselves. People discover through mindfulness practice (Oken *et al.* 2010)[2] that perceived stress levels can decrease and they feel better (see page 149).

Sometimes talking things through with other family carers or support organisations can alleviate the stress. Family carers have identified the following needs:

- talking to someone who understands and who will listen

- learning how to deal with changes caused by dementia

- learning how to deal with changes in the relationship

- learning how to cope with stress so I stay well

- learning how to help my relative live more meaningfully

- learning about different options for end-of-life care

- knowing where to go for advice and support on legal matters; state support; physical support

- knowing where the dementia-friendly places are.

Emotional support can be the mainstay in enabling people to regain a sense of resilience and purpose. The nature of relationships does change, but it does not have to be a negative experience. People discover aspects of themselves and the other that they would otherwise have never known. The relationship can remain two-way, even though the communication may need to change.

Quality of life and care is highly dependent on the quality of relationship between the caregiver and care recipient. That is quite a responsibility. Many care staff are only just beginning to appreciate the importance of connecting with people, although the concept of therapeutic relationship has been around for decades. When we talk about person-centred care in care facilitates, we are also referring to quality of relationships.

Buber (2000)[3] suggests a person grows through relationship with others, especially when affirmed in his or her wholeness.

We can do that by fully acknowledging the presence of a person and validating them as a whole human being, rather than regarding them as someone incomplete or in need of fixing. A deeper relationship develops when we practice being more open in our perceptions. This allows us to see the person's qualities, which feels affirming and liberating.

McCance, MacCormack and Dewing (2011)[4] emphasise the importance of relationships and the therapeutic effect they can have. They argue that person-centred nursing involves being in relation, being in a social world, being in place, and being with self. Person-centredness is 'multi-dimensional' and needs relationships built on mutual trust, understanding and sharing of knowledge.

People involved in giving and receiving care are in complex relationship with each other as well as with the disease or illness and the organisations concerned. There is often a parallel process in terms of individual needs or experiences. For example, each person may be seeking reassurance. The person being cared for wants to know they are in safe hands. The person doing the caring wants to know that they are doing the right thing.

Research quoted in Nolan *et al.*'s 2004 article (Davies *et al.* 1999; Nolan 1997; Nolan *et al.*, 2001, 2002) led to a 'senses framework' that supports everyone involved in caring relationships by promoting a sense of security, belonging, continuity, purpose, achievement and significance.

Each person will need support at different times and in different ways. Some carers and people living with dementia lose their sense of belonging to the wider society. Dementia cafes, singing groups, creative workshops, library talks and befrienders can all help people to feel more connected.

Activities, such as the life-story books or stargazing can support a sense of belonging and continuity on the personal level as well as in the universal scheme of things. Activities that feel meaningful and accessible support a sense of purpose and satisfaction. It is important to understand the ways in which people living with dementia may experience the world. But equally essential is understanding that his or her sense of value is affected by the perceptions and responses of others. We can all be more aware of this.

Activities to support relationships

Many of the activities in this book support relationships by helping people to interact in ways that do not focus on dementia. The following activities are for family carers and care staff to do, as well people living with dementia and care staff.

MAP-MAKING

The metaphor of a map is perfect for supporting people to describe where they feel they are at emotionally, socially and mentally. We use this with family carers just as much as with people living with dementia. The map offers reference points that help people see their journey so far, and offers an opportunity to add new routes.

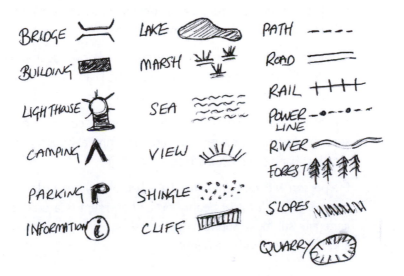

Figure 3.1: Map legend

As with any map, the experience of walking the terrain is different to the representation, but many people have found this a useful tool. We begin by looking at maps, usually of the area most familiar to the person, which could be in the past, or a current location.

Talk about the contours, look up the map legend for viewpoints, outcrops, marshland, cliff edges, woodland, etc. Use magnifying glasses or sheets to aid sight. You can print map legends from the Internet.

Take a look at a mapping model called 'the journey of becoming reconnected' (Marshall 2013),[6] shown below, that describes a process experienced by caregivers and care recipients living with the diagnosis and effects of dementia; the stages may include the following:

○ intimacy – the comfort and familiarity of life before the illness

○ dawning – recognising that things are not quite right, but mostly able to explain things away as a phase, or stress, etc.

○ holding on – changes become more noticeable, but it is the big battle for independence and keeping things as normal as possible. Can be a period of great tension

○ letting go – the point at which there may be acknowledgement of the illness (sometimes only by the caregiver), and sometimes a recognition of need for respite

○ alienation – the next part of the journey becomes more separate for the caregiver and care recipient, although they may be sharing the same space

○ the person with dementia may have hills or abysses, but they may also find places of beauty or 'wonderment'. Carers are generally still busy supporting themselves, the household, and the person with dementia

○ support – the carer and/or the person with dementia may seek support and information, or the support may be made more clearly available

○ inner work – the carer often goes on an inner journey that may include working through feelings of loss, anger and guilt, as well as feelings of relief, love and peace. This inner work is about self-discovery. The carer recognises that he or she is a person besides being a carer, and a person besides being a wife, husband, son or daughter. The caregiver allows the relationship to change. This is one of the most difficult transitions to make

○ wonderment – these are the spaces and times when the caregiver and care-recipient experience connection through 'wonderment'…something joyful, such as singing, creative activities or being in nature

○ reconnection – this is not the same as the intimacy in the beginning. It is beyond the personal, and in 'the-moment-of-now'. There may be no recognition, but the feeling of connection is still real and valid.

Carers and people in early to mid-stages of dementia generally recognise these stages. Typically, when people do this activity, they are just past the middle of the process – around the support and inner work stage. The next set of questions supports people in creating the map. Individuals can choose which stages they wish to represent and which symbols to use.

1. How did the landscape look at the initial signs of illness?

2. What sort of ground did you feel you were on?

3. As you became clearer about the illness, did the landscape change (was it easier/more difficult)?

4. Do you feel your paths have diverged, or are you still walking together?

5. What bridges of support or information points are available to you?

6. What terrain would you like there to be in front of you?

7. What would places of wonderment look like to you?

The maps are sometimes coded and difficult for anyone except the map-maker to understand. This indicates an important need for privacy, and should be respected. Sometimes people openly share their map, and keep it as a record of how far they have travelled. During discussions some family carers have not been able to imagine a place of wonderment. However, after a few weeks, sometimes months, they have been surprised to find that there is a place for wonderment and reconnection on their maps.

TALKING HEADS

This is a more light-hearted and humorous activity and is again done with people in early to mid-stages of dementia. The task is to create silhouettes with moving mouthpieces that can 'speak' to each other. This is usually done as a shadow-puppet, and requires a third person so that people can take turns in observing the activity. The activity can also be done with two people, without the shadow screens. You will need paper, pencil, cardboard, scissors, a paper-fastener and an optional stick or tightly rolled-up magazine page.

To create a silhouette of someone's head you could ask them to sit sideways on, near a window, so that you can see their outline more clearly. Draw the outline as near to life size as possible, onto some paper.

Another option is to fix some white paper on the wall behind the person, who sits in profile. Shine a lamp to cast a shadow of their head onto the paper. Draw around the outline of the shadow; include details that can seen, such as eyelashes or hair that sticks up (Step 1 in Figure 3.2). Then swap places if possible, so that you are now the sitter for the artist.

If these practicalities seem too difficult, a third option is to take photographs of the profile of each person's head and have these enlarged.

Whichever process you use, you should have two heads. Glue these onto cardboard and cut around the image outlines.

To create a moving mouth, take another piece of card and place it beneath the bottom part of your head, level with the bottom lip. Trace round the bottom part of the head onto the card, then remove the card and on the new part that you have just drawn, mark a sloping line from the lips to about 1cm higher at the back of the head.

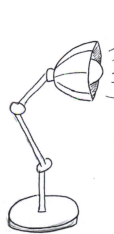
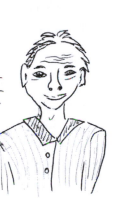
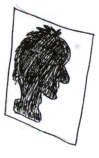

Step 1

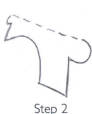
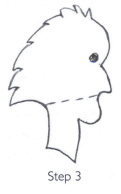
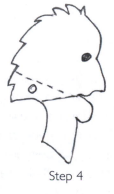

Step 2   Step 3   Step 4

Figure 3.2: Making a 'talking head'

Cut out the new shape (Step 2 in Figure 3.2). Now draw a sloping line on the main head from the middle of the lips sloping gradually by 1cm down to the back of the head. Cut along the line (Step 3). Now fix the new part of the head to the original head, using the paper fastener, so that the bottom jaw (the whole lower part of the head in this instance) is free to move up and down (Step 4).

When both heads are done, they are ready to start talking! Choose any topic and see what happens. Try casting the shadows of the heads onto a wall or ceiling, so that you see the effects more clearly. The effects can be very funny.

BREATHING TOGETHER

It is important to find ways of being with someone in comfortable silence. The practice of communicating this way becomes more valuable in later stages of dementia. People do not need to be bombarded by words or sounds. The following two activities are about communicating love and respect without needing to say anything.

Breathing together requires a quiet room and about three to ten minutes of undisturbed time. With practice this activity can be extended, but initially it is usually better to keep it brief.

Offer a verbal invitation to sit together in silence. Offer to rearrange cushions or pillows, etc., so that the person is in a comfortable position, and do the same for yourself. Uncross crossed limbs, and feel yourself fully supported by the chair or bed or floor.

After 30 seconds or so, become more focused on the breathing, breathing in through the nose and out through the mouth. You could watch and listen to how the person you support is breathing. Sometimes you can match their breathing and then purposefully slow your own breathing down. The person may follow your lead, deepening their breath as they relax. (It is of no matter if they do not do this.)

As you become more relaxed, look at the face of the person you are supporting. Notice the physical features, the shape of the face, the eyes, nose and mouth. Notice the colour and markings of the skin. Consider all the years this face has lived and what this face has witnessed. Wonder about the tears and laughter this face has expressed and all the happy birthdays it has known. Now send thoughts of love and appreciation to this person who is in connection with you by simply being there.

Take a few moments to refocus your attention back into the room. This is an activity that can build the relationships in a different way...sometimes a deeper way. There is more about breathing activities in Chapter 4.

HAND STUDY

You may want to use hand cream or just gentle touch for this activity. You could go so far as soaking the hands in a bowl of warm water and drying them before applying hand cream, so that the experience is more like a manicure.

Take the person's hand in a gentle and comfortable way and compare it to your own. There is no need to speak. Just hold your hand against their hand, noticing differences in size, shape or colour. Look at the person's palm. See the lines that have been changing throughout their lives. Are the lines deep or faint? Do they have a chain effect pattern? Broken lines? Can you see any star shapes in the palm?

Consider whose hands these hands have held. Consider the work these hands have done. Sit holding hands in wonderment about these things.

PEG WEAVING

This activity is so lovely to share together, and accessible to people who may have only limited physical dexterity. However, it does require a simple peg loom and materials prepared in advance. You can create colourful wall-hangings or table mats, using wool and threading on beads or tying in ribbons.

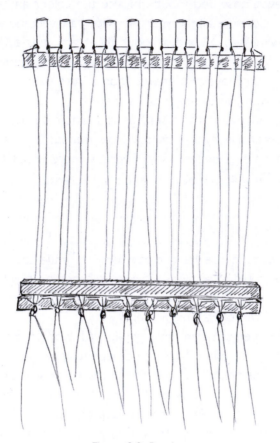

Figure 3.3: Peg loom

The pegs along the loom determine the width of the piece, and the length is determined by how long you decide to make the strings (the warp threads) from the pegs upon which the weaving moves down.

Decide on the length of your weaving, and cut pieces of thread that are double that length. Thread each peg with the doubled length of string or wool, until the middle of the thread is in the peg. Tie a knot at the end of each pair of peg strings. It is safer to tie these again to the neighbouring peg strings, or clip them all together, so your weave does not slip off the ends.

The weave works on a flat surface as well as on the edge of a table…depending on how far a person's hand can reach.

Tie your first strand of wool (start either end of the peg-loom) to an end peg. Not too tightly, as the whole weave needs to be free to move down the warp threads.

Weave the wool in and out of the pegs, passing the wool in front, and behind alternate pegs. If you want beads or objects in the weave, tie off the wool at the end of the row and cut it. Thread a new piece of wool with the beads, and then tie this to where you left off before. You can move beads into position as you continue weaving. Keep going, adding more wool until the pegs are almost full.

Now lift the first peg and push the wool down along the strings. Do this for each peg, replacing them in their holes. Continue weaving until you have reached your desired length. Now push the wool along its strings, making sure the weave is as tight as you would like. Cut the strings off the first two pegs and tie into a knot close to the weave. Do the same with each pair of pegs. Check all knots are secure.

The weavings could be done using colours of the seasons, which look very effective. One care setting did a group weaving to hang in their home.

SOMETHING COMPLETELY DIFFERENT

This activity does exactly what it is called. You and the person are challenged to do something completely different to get a new perspective. Sit under a table; lie on the floor; eat with your non-dominant hand…anything that is unusual. Some people do not like changes to routine, but it can depend on how it is done and whether the fun of something feels better than the routine. Do what feels right. Try something different once a week or so. It does not have to be a physical activity – it could be learning a new word or trying a new food.

Interacting in creative and interesting ways helps build good relationships.

References

1. Crocker, J. and Garcia, J. (2009) 'Downward and Upward Spirals in Intergroup Interactions: The Role of Egosystem and Ecosystem Goals.' In T.D. Nelson (ed.) *Handbook of Prejudice, Stereotyping, and Discrimination.* New York: Psychology Press, p.240.

2. Oken, B.S., Fonareva, I., Haas, M., Wahbeh, H., Lane, J.B., Zajdel, D., and Amen, A. (2010). 'Pilot controlled trial of mindfulness meditation and education for dementia caregivers.' *Journal of Alternative and Complementary Medicine 16*, 10, 1031–1038. doi:10.1089/acm.2009.0733. Available at www.ncbi.nlm.nih.gov/pmc/articles/PMC3110802. Accessed on 14 August 2015.

3. Buber, M. (2000). 'I and Thou' (1958). Translated by Ronald Gregor Smith. London: Simon & Schuster.

4. McCance, T., McCormack, B. and Dewing, J. (2011) 'An Exploration of Person-Centredness in Practice.' *The Online Journal of Issues in Nursing 16*, 2, manuscript 1. doi: 10.3912/OJIN.Vol16No02Man01. Available at www.nursingworld.org/MainMenuCategories/ANAMarketplace/ ANAPeriodicals/OJIN/TableofContents/Vol-16-2011/No2-May-2011/ Person-Centredness-in-Practice.html. Accessed on 14 August 2015.

5. Nolan, M., Davies, S., Brown, J., Keady, J. and Nolan, J. (2004). 'Beyond 'person-centred' care: A new vision for gerontological nursing.' *International Journal of Older People Nursing* [in association with the *Journal of Clinical Nursing*] *13*, 3a, 45–53.

6. Marshall, K. *Puppetry in Dementia Care: Connecting through Creativity and Joy.* London and Philadelphia, PA: Jessica Kingsley Publishers.

Resources

Peg loom stockist: Creativity in Care™. See www.creativityincare.org for details of prices and delivery charges.

◦ 4 ◦

SUPPORTING PHYSICAL HEALTH

Physical health is one of the more quantifiably measurable outcomes in holistic care. Whilst some people may consider good physical health to mean freedom from disease, it has a much wider definition, and includes various degrees of fitness and health (with and without disease). The benefits of physical health also increase emotional wellbeing and alertness.

Our physical health can be measured in terms of physical activity, muscle strength, body flexibility, body mass index (BMI) and weight, breath flow, cholesterol levels, blood sugar levels, blood pressure, quality of sleep, nutrition, fluid intake and output, bowel movement, alcohol consumption, pain levels and medication. These measures show the range of factors involved in maintaining physical health.

We make lifestyle choices regarding what we eat, when we sleep or how much exercise we take. People who live independently have more control over these choices, but not everyone follows the healthy recommendations. Several papers have been written about the problem of 'non-adherence' to advice about lifestyle change (or to medical advice). It appears that most of us do not stick to health recommendations.

Martin *et al.* (2005)[1] looked at why there is a low take-up of advice, and found a range of key factors to improve adherence to suggested lifestyle changes. A major factor is to ensure that communication is effective, so that information and suggestions are clear and understandable. This becomes even more important if the person has disease affecting memory or comprehension.

Getting to know what matters to the person is an essential factor. There is little point in making lots of healthy suggestions if the person feels far removed from such possibilities. Sometimes attitudes and beliefs are barriers to adherence. People may not believe the advice will make any difference. They may feel there is little point to health routines, when they have a terminal illness. Depression significantly reduces people's motivation for self-care.

Hall *et al.* (1996)[2] reflected that the health of a person affected how physicians behaved towards them. There is a tendency to be more negative around people who are ill or distressed…and this only compounds the issues. As carers, our relationships with people living with dementia and other conditions, matter greatly. Through relationship we can build trust.

Hoffman (2013)[3] claims that we tend to listen to advice from celebrities. He suggests that this is because they are regarded as trustworthy, even though they may be speaking about factors outside their area of expertise. The point here is that we need to build that kind of emotional connection and trust.

When we feel a connection with the advice, or to the source of the advice, we are more likely to follow it. Our relationships and emotional wellbeing influence our willingness to give things a go. Physical health relies on feeling motivated enough to bother. By understanding what matters to individuals, we can find ways to help people understand the benefits of physical health. We can make things feel more interesting and relevant, and a part of everyday life.

Physical activity – warnings about inactivity

Most of us are aware of the importance of physical exercise. There are vast quantities of media articles, books, CDs, DVDs, magazines, TV programmes and community fitness classes highlighting the benefits of physical activity. Even so, there is growing concern about our sedentary lifestyles (sitting at computers or watching TV, driving everywhere or sitting in meetings).

In 2006 the World Health Organisation for Europe called upon national, regional and local governments to help tackle the challenge of sedentary living. We know that in care homes and hospitals people sit for long periods of the day.

Research by Nicolai et al. (2010)[4] found that nursing home residents spend 80 to 90 per cent of their time seated or in bed. One week of bed rest reduces leg strength by 20 per cent. Some people are seated or resting because of pain or illness or fear of falling – yet movement and balance exercises can alleviate these symptoms. The majority of people are sedentary because of lack of opportunity or motivation.

Other researchers in sedentary and physical activities, Henson et al. (2013),[5] involved almost 800,000 participants from around the world. There were clear associations between sedentary behaviour and health risks. They looked at the health differences between people who sat the least and sat the most, and found that those who sat the most have:

- 147 per cent increased risk of cardiovascular events

- 112 per cent increased risk of diabetes

- 90 per cent increased risk of cardiovascular mortality

- 49 per cent increased risk of all-cause mortality.

Lack of movement can lead to physical and mental difficulties, such as bowel problems, digestion issues, boredom and depression. Sitting for long periods affects the body's ability to maintain balanced blood sugar levels and blood pressure.

In 2011, a report called *Start Active, Stay Active* by four chief medical officers for Scotland, England, Wales and Northern Ireland[6] highlighted further problems of sedentary behaviour:

> Older adults, particularly those who are inactive, are susceptible to a loss of muscle mass and a reduction in bone density as well as increased body fat. Loss of muscle strength accompanied by carrying large amounts of excess fat will contribute to decreased function and mobility, making it more difficult to achieve simple tasks such as getting out of chairs and walking up stairs and slopes. Loss of muscle strength and being underweight can also impair an individual's ability to undertake daily tasks.
>
> (DoH 2011, p.42)

Physical inactivity is identified as the fourth leading risk factor for death in the world. It is estimated by the World Health Organisation (WHO 2011)[7] to be the main cause of approximately 21–25 per cent of breast and colon cancers, 27 per cent of diabetes and approximately 30 per cent of transient ischaemic attack (TIA). As cardiovascular diseases are the leading cause of death in the world, it is clear that we need to promote the benefits of physical activity.

Benefits of physical exercise

First, any increase in physical exercise offers benefits. Even if we do not see changes in body weight and shape, we still experience health gains. Regular physical activity helps to reduce risks of type 2 diabetes, cancer, obesity, coronary heart disease and stroke. Exercise increases the flow of oxygen to the brain. Our brains use 20 per cent of the body's oxygen to function, so it is important to support the flow of blood that carries oxygen, especially if brain disease is present.

There is much evidence to support the positive impact of exercise on balance and preventing falls. Falls are a major cause of injury for older adults. People living with later stages of dementia may also be susceptible to falls due to impaired balance, eyesight or perception problems, and muscle weakness from inactivity. Balance training and muscle strengthening activities help to reduce the risk of falls.

Physical activity increases our sense of general wellbeing and life satisfaction. People who do some physical movement (e.g. through creative activity, dance or walking) comment on feeling better and more alive, even whilst living with the more advanced symptoms of dementia.

Group exercises in community or care settings, or shared exercises at home with family members can help people feel more socially included. Alzheimer Australia NSW's discussion paper (2014)[8] reports better communication and alertness following exercise:

> People with dementia and carers reported the physical benefits, including feeling stronger, improvements in coordination and balance, and general sense of wellbeing as a result of remaining physically active and exercising. Some also felt that there were cognitive benefits, including a potential correlation between the presentation and progression of dementia and a physically active lifestyle. People with dementia and family members noted that they or the person they support are more alert and communicate more effectively on days they are more physically active.
>
> (Alzheimer Australia NSW 2014)

So, given that we know the risks of inactivity and the benefits of activity, how do we find ways to motivate people to do physical activity? First, by being clear ourselves about the risks and benefits, so that we can communicate these to others. Next we need to understand recommended guidelines.

What are the recommended guidelines for activity in adults and older adults?

The WHO *Global Recommendations on Physical Activity for Health* (2011)[7] and the UK *Start Active, Stay Active* guidelines (2011)[6] show the importance of regular exercise. Several short sessions of activity for about 10 minutes seem to be as effective as (and in some cases more effective than) sitting all day with one longer burst of activity.

1. Exercise needs to be regular, but any exercise is better than none.

2. People should aim to be active daily and achieve 150 minutes (2.5 hours) of moderate intensity activity every week. This could be done in bouts of 10 minutes or more.

3. People who are already regularly active at *moderate* intensity can gain benefit from 75 minutes of *vigorous* intensity activity per week (or a combination of moderate and vigorous activity).

4. Older adults should also undertake physical activity to improve muscle strength on at least two days a week. Performing 8–12 repetitions of muscle strengthening activities involving all major muscle groups will provide substantial benefits for older adults.

5. Adults at risk of falls should incorporate physical activity to improve balance and co-ordination on at least two days a week.

6. All adults should minimise the amount of time spent sitting for extended periods.

The rates at which we expend energy vary depending on our levels of fitness and experience of illness, to begin with. For some people, the effort of moving from a chair to a bed can feel huge, so the following levels of activity intensity are very general.

1. *Sedentary* behaviour expends very little energy – for example, watching TV, sleeping, resting, reading, travelling by road or rail, studying or working at the computer, having seated meetings and chats.

2. *Low to moderate intensity* activity raises the heart rate. People may break into a sweat, but still be able to hold a conversation while exercising. This includes leisurely swimming, gardening, leisure dancing, chair exercises, household cleaning, carrying shopping, walking, some cycling and aerobic exercises.

3. *Vigorous intensity* activity raises the heart rate further. People usually sweat and their breathing is hard and fast. Activities include competitive swimming, jogging, gym workouts, and more aerobic activities.

For people who have very low levels of physical activity, shorter periods of exercise may feel more achievable. Any exercise is better than none. Even standing up from a sitting position every hour will benefit circulation and health. We have noticed more risk factors in sedentary living than in exercise, but it is important to consider activity-related risk. Small and gradual increases in activity suited to each individual will minimise such risks. It is advisable to seek the support of a physical activities or medical practitioner to help plan a suitable programme.

Making exercise relevant, meaningful or fun

The following activities support physical health for being active, getting fresh air, stimulating the brain, maintaining balance, eating and sleeping well. They have been used with individuals and groups living with dementia, as well as people with interested in creative ways of feeling more physically healthy. Changes in a person's usual routine may need to be planned for, and assessed or monitored by the individual or carer. (See more about managing risk on pages 185–186.)

We know that clear communication and support from trusted advisors help people engage with healthy life activities. The following factors also help:

- the person's belief that he or she is capable of doing things (self-efficacy)

- feeling interested or inspired by the topic or event

- having opportunities to try things.

It is important that carers engage with the activities too, otherwise it will be difficult to convey any sense of enthusiasm or genuine support. The activities benefit everyone involved, but as we are all unique, choose the ones that feel best to you and the person you support.

BIRD-WATCHING

Whilst bird-watching can happen from the comfort of a chair or bed, it has even more benefits when we go outside. The brain benefits from fresh air and daylight. Daylight through our eyes stimulates the brain's setting of the biological or circadian clock in the hypothalamus. The hypothalamus is about the size of an almond nut and sits just above the brain stem. It helps to maintain systems such as sleep cycles, hunger and thirst, heart rate and body temperature.

Going out to look for birds makes the physical exercise more pleasurable and interesting. Even putting food out daily offers an opportunity to be physically active. Learning about birds (identifying them, learning their songs and understanding their behaviour) stimulates the brain to create new neural pathways.

There are bird-watching organisations around the world with advice and tips on what to look for. Binoculars are not essential, but can be very useful. Sometimes having a sheet of the most likely birds to be seen is easier for people to cope with than a whole book of bird images.

Initially people regard all birds as something with a head, a body, a beak, two wings and two feet. However, with practised looking, people learn to recognise the basic body parts that give more clues to identification.

TYPES OF BEAK:

- ○ small and stout beak – seed-eating birds, such as sparrows and chaffinches
- ○ small and pointed break – insect-catching birds, such as swallows
- ○ flat beak – ducks
- ○ large and hooked beak – birds of prey, such as falcons
- ○ sharp beak – crows that eat a wide range of things
- ○ long and pointed beak – can be for probing flowers for nectar
- ○ long beak – can be used for fishing or opening shellfish (e.g. oyster catchers).

Take a pen and notebook to keep a log-book of the birds spotted. On occasion these notebooks have become weather records and stimulated an interest in drawing different cloud shapes. The bird-watching can easily lead to other interests, but it is a particular passtime that many people are devoted to. Some people enjoy taking a camera and using the opportunity to photograph nature. Look for photographic competitions online or in local newspapers for opportunities to enter photos.

Check the following organisations for advice and information sheets. Even reading about birds from around the world can inspire topics of conversation. Imagine, in Scotland, being able to attract parrots into your garden; or spot a tufted flycatcher from America, or see grouse in Australia.

○ Britain: The Royal Society for the Protection of Birds

   www.rspb.org.uk

○ Australia: The Birdlife Organisation

   www.birdlife.org.au

○ America: The American Birding Association

   www.aba.org

○ Japan: Wild Bird Society Japan

   www.wbsj.org

CHANNELING ANDY GOLDSWORTHY

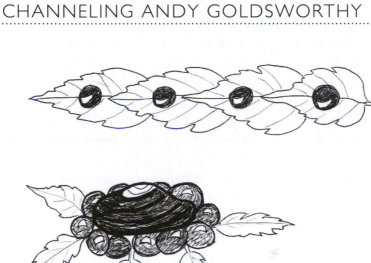

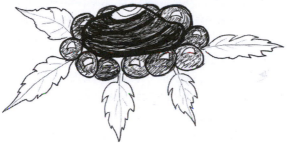

Figure 4.1: Leaves and berries

A favourite activity is creating patterns or sculptures from natural materials and allowing them to be washed or blown away by the elements. Andy Goldsworthy is a British artist and sculptor who has created artworks around the world, including Japan, America, and Australia. You can do this activity with groups in woodlands and beaches or in the garden.

Benefits include getting fresh air and daylight, combined with physical activity for finding natural materials to work with. The amount of daylight we get can affect our mood. Many people experience seasonal affective disorder (SAD) in the winter months in northern countries. In Alaska it is estimated that one in ten people are affected and feel depressed or lethargic. Being outside in daylight is an important part of physical health.

If mobility for bending down is an issue, it can be useful to prepare a camping table. The person can work with materials gathered by more flexible people, on a piece of cardboard or hardboard.

To begin with, it is usually helpful to show images of the artwork created by Andy Goldsworthy from his books.[9,10] Ask people for ideas of shapes to create on the ground or on the board. Spirals and hearts are popular, but the shape could be as simple as a squiggly line or an oval. These can serve as reminders if required later when it comes to making the art.

Take hand wipes or thin rubber gloves for people handling natural materials. Only use materials that are on the ground or already free from their original plant, so that no damage is done to living trees, shrubs and flowers.

Collect pine needles, twigs, pebbles, leaves, petals and seeds.

Create the patterns. Pine needles can be used to pin leaves together, or water can temporarily stick petals to pebbles. Take photos of the patterns being created. This is a creative activity that has no right or wrong about it…and people enjoy doing this several times, as it is different each time.

The activity could be extended to creating mosaic patterns set in plaster of Paris or cement mortar, or with strong glue and grouting. Use shells, pebbles and mosaic squares. The work does not require speech or memory…People can stick pieces into ready-drawn patterns, or just work within a defined space to do whatever they want.

Mosaic projects are ideal for group work and make attractive garden features when set into the ground or as a wall hanging.

STAR-GAZING

While daylight is important, there is something very exciting and mysterious about going out during the night. The benefits include fresh air and stimulation and a sense of something special. Not many people get the chance to step outside and see the moon or stars, yet it is such a beautiful activity to do…even just once a year.

Having the opportunity to focus on something in the distance is also good exercise for the eyes.

Ensure that people are wrapped up warm and have areas to sit when needed. Poor light affects mobility in many people, so allow plenty of time for walking to the seated area, with gentle verbal or physical guidance if required. If the area you live in has a lot of light pollution, focus on looking at the moon. Check which phase of the moon cycle we are in (waxing, full or waning). The moon reflects light from the sun and we see different parts of it lit up, although we always see the same side of the moon. It is possible to see some of the moon's landscape…

The ideal conditions for stargazing are on a moonless, clear night. However, it is still possible to make out a few stars between clouds and even when the moon is bright. Stargazing puts things into perspective. We contemplate the universe and recognise how much there is yet to learn and understand. This great unknown is in harmony with all the other great unknowns about brain disease and wellness.

One of the men we worked with talked with some satisfaction about his experience of dementia. He said he could see the stars through the holes in his mind. This led to a discussion about being made up of stardust and the enormity of the universe.

People do not need words or memory to feel the magnificence of a starry night. Allow plenty of time for people to settle into the activity. We find it helpful to give clues about what the activity is about. Show images of the moon and stars in books, or a print of Van Gogh's starry night.

Sing songs about the stars and space: 'Starry, starry night' by Don McLean; 'Space oddity' by David Bowie; 'Rocket man' by Elton John; 'Would you like to swing on a star?' and 'Fly me to the moon' by Frank Sinatra.

There are many references to the night sky and space in fiction and non-fiction books that can add to the event. In the novel *Contact* by Carl Sagan (1985),[9] a girl watches the stars while contemplating how the universe works:

The sky was blazing with stars. There were thousands of them, most twinkling, a few bright and steady, If you looked carefully you could see faint differences in colour. That bright one there. Wasn't it bluish? … At one end of the sky the stars were rising. That way was called East. At the other end of the sky, behind her, beyond the cabins, the stars were setting. That way was called West. Once every day the Earth would spin completely around, and the same stars would rise again in the same place.

> (Reprinted with the permission of Little, Brown Book Group and Simon & Schuster, Inc. from *Contact* by Carl Sagan © 1985 Carl Sagan)

In his epic poem *Evangeline: A Tale of Acadie*[12] Henry Wadsworth Longfellow describes a beautiful and romantic night sky:

> Meanwhile apart, in the twilight gloom of a window's embrasure,
> Sat the lovers, and whispered together, beholding the moon rise
> Over the pallid sea and the silvery mist of the meadows.
> Silently one by one, in the infinite meadows of heaven,
> Blossomed the lovely stars, the forget-me-nots of the angels.
>
> (Longfellow 1847)

WHAT TO LOOK FOR IN THE NIGHT SKY:

Before tilting the head back, do some gentle shoulder-raising and -lowering warm-up movements. Cradle the back of the neck between the shoulders and gently roll it from side to side. Make sure there is a chair back or some support before asking people to look up, in case anyone becomes unsteady. Allow people time to lift their heads as much as feels comfortable. We usually concentrate on looking for around ten minutes, with some chatter and occasionally a flask of warm milk.

Most of the stargazing can be done using your eyes, but occasionally using binoculars. It is easier to hold a steady gaze with our eyes. There are some star patterns or constellations that most people will have heard of. In the northern hemisphere, the North Star is usually visible. It is in a relatively fixed position in the sky, aligned with earth's spinning axis. All other stars revolve around this star.

If you can see the following you have made a great start:

○ The Plough (UK) or The Big Dipper (US)

○ The North Star (also currently Polaris or polar star)

○ Cassiopeia, the great W shape.

On some nights it is possible to see planets. Our brightest planets are Venus, Mars, Mercury, Jupiter and Saturn.

In the southern hemisphere (oceans and countries south of the Equator) there is not such a bright star as the North Star, but there are more visible stars of the Milky Way, including a small distant galaxy orbiting our galaxy. Stargazers also get to see the well-known Southern Cross (or Crux). Star maps or charts can be found on the numerous websites dedicated to astronomy.

Indoor energy exercises

BREATHING AND BALANCE

Because balance is such an integral part of any activity, people usually understand the importance of improving their balance. Some exercises for people recovering from stroke are also used for people in later stages of dementia.

Before undertaking any exercise, allow time for the body to relax and prepare itself. We usually begin with a breathing exercise.

Sit comfortably on a chair that has arms, with both feet resting on the floor or supported on a footstool – or in bed, with pillows to support you sitting up.

If it is possible, place one hand on your chest and one on your abdomen, whilst breathing normally. (This breathing exercise can still be done without the hands being involved.)

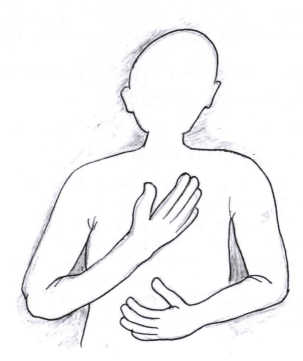

Figure 4.2: Breathing

After a minute or so, become more focused on your breathing... breathing in through your nose and out through your mouth. On the next inbreath allow the breath to come deeply into your body, so that the abdomen swells. (The hand on the abdomen feels this expansion.) On the outbreath, the abdomen decreases. This movement means that the diaphragm is moving down on the inbreath, and up on the outbreath. It is a form of deep breathing that most animals use when in a state of relaxation. As you do this for two or three times, the muscles begin to relax and the breathing exercise is beneficial just as it is.

The sitting balance is a set of gentle movements that move the upper half of the upper body from side to side, and forwards and backwards. For the side-to-side movement, we are focused on moving the ribcage only. It takes practice, but the idea is to shift weight first onto one hip, then onto the other, by shifting the ribcage each way. (If we bend at the waist we are not really shifting the weight.)

If you can hold the sides of the chair you can feel the weight first in one arm, then in the other arm, which helps the arm muscles. If you are sitting on a bench, use books to rest your hands on. Do this five to ten times at regular intervals throughout the day.

For the forward and backward motion, do this very gently. This movement happens by rounding the back slightly to bring the ribcage backwards, and arching the back slightly to bring the ribcage forward. You can feel this small movement engaging stomach and back muscles as well. Do this five to ten times at regular intervals throughout the day.

CHAIR MARCHING

This is an effective exercise for balance, alertness and fitness. It is sometimes called 'cross-crawling' and is used as a Brain Gym exercise because it stimulates the sensory motor area and central nervous system. This contralateral movement is something babies learn to do when crawling, and helps connect the two hemispheres of the brain, for better flow of information. If we have been sedentary or unwell, this movement may take a little practice to become re-established.

Whilst it is good to do this as a standing exercise, it works well in a seated position too. The exercise involves lifting one arm and the opposite leg together, then changing to the other arm and opposite leg, in a marching fashion. Even small movements will work. It is better to march slowly and to stop if there is any sign of tiredness or pain. As with all exercise, it is important to build strength and body patterns gradually and slowly. The movement strengthens leg and arm muscles as well as balance.

This exercise can be varied to add interest and challenge, but remember to keep it a steady, slow movement.

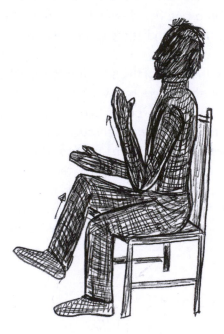

Figure 4.3: Chair marching

1. Lift one arm out to the side when opposite knee is raised, and then the other arm to the other side for the opposite knee.
2. With one arm and the opposite leg, reach out on a diagonal line, whilst bringing the other arm and leg inwards. Then swap sides.

BED MARCHING

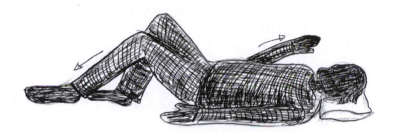

Figure 4.4: Bed marching

Another version of cross-crawling can be done whilst lying on the bed with raised knees:

1. First, with knees bent, do some breathing (see the 'Breathing and balance' section). Only do what feels comfortable.
2. On each outbreath, allow your lower back to sink gradually into the bed. Do not force this. Have your arms loosely by your sides.
3. When you are ready, on the next outbreath, lower one knee, so that the leg stretches. Breathe in (rest).
4. Breathe out (rest)…
5. and on the next inbreath, gradually raise the knee again.
6. Repeat with the other leg.

If that feels comfortable, repeat three or four times.

If still comfortable, you can then involve the arms:

Begin with simple movements. Keep your shoulders and elbows on the bed.

1. Breathe in.
2. Breathe out, and as you lower your left knee and stretch your left leg, raise your right hand and forearm, so that your hand comes back towards your shoulder.
3. Breathe in (rest).
4. Breathe out (rest).
5. On the next inbreath raise your knee and lower your hand and forearm.
6. Repeat with your right leg and left hand.

Rest in between movements. If your arms, shoulders and ribs feel well, you could try lifting the whole arm backwards to stretch behind your head. But only do this if it feels comfortable, and keep your shoulders on the bed. The simpler movements are still stimulating the brain.

Cross-crawling can be done as a daily exercise and is relatively easy to build into the daily routine. You can march whilst on your way to the bathroom, or whilst sitting in a chair. People notice that they feel more awake as a result. One man commented that he knew his army training would come in useful one day.

Eating

In care settings, or even at home, a day may revolve around mealtimes. Meals take on greater significance in a day when there is less stimulation. Many people say they look forward to mealtimes. These times give meaning to the day. It is therefore easy to see why food presentation and taste matter.

Changes in eating habits are common with age or when living with long-term conditions. If people eat alone it can be hard for them to feel motivated enough to cook for themselves. Some families cook extra portions for their relative to heat up during the week. Use labels and clear instructions to support independence. Befriending schemes can help by people sharing a meal together. Others may need to use meal delivery programmes.

Certain food aromas can stimulate appetite. Cinnamon spice sprinkled on toast or coffee smells good. Many people enjoy the aroma of fried onion, sizzling bacon, fresh bread and roast chicken. Our preferences are very individual, so see which food smells are most liked.

Loss of appetite, particularly in later stages of dementia, is a common cause of concern for family carers and care staff. It can be caused by physical, emotional, cognitive and/or environmental issues…but it does not always indicate a major problem. As long as people are still getting the right nutrients, a decrease in portion size is OK. Sometimes eating little and often is preferable.

Nutrients should include proteins, calcium, B vitamins and fibre. Typically these include foods such as tuna fish, salmon and mackerel, cheese, milk, eggs (or non-dairy substitutes), fruit and vegetables, wholemeal bread, cereals, grains and nuts. If extra calories are needed, use some olive oil, peanut butter, avocado, or powdered milk.

Before making any change it is worth sitting with the person and a medical practitioner who can help assess the best way forward. Some neurological disorders can affect the muscles involved in swallowing and digestion. There are several possible causes for appetite changes. The following questions or observations can help the physician/medical advisor to understand what is going on.

1. Is this a sudden change in appetite or a gradual decline?

2. Has it ever happened before (and if so, what were the circumstances)?

3. Have eating patterns or times changed? In what ways?

4. Has the person's weight changed?

5. Is the person experiencing stress or anxiety?

6. Is it difficult for the person to chew food?

7. How well does the mouth look?

8. Does the person have signs of tooth decay?

9. Do dentures fit properly?

10. Is it difficult for the person to swallow food?

11. Is there any pain when they swallow?

12. Does the person experience choking when eating or drinking (and if so, does this happen regularly or rarely)?

13. Does the person complain of food sticking in their throat? Or in their chest?

14. Do they have an excessive cough?

15. Do they regurgitate food? Does this happen through the nose?

16. Does the person's breath smell (halitosis)?

17. Is there excessive saliva?

18. Does the person have chest pain after eating?

19. Do they need to burp a lot after eating?

20. Does the person experience acid reflux (stomach acid coming back up into the mouth)?

21. What sorts of foods make this worse?

22. Which foods appear to cause bloating?

23. If indigestion or heartburn is experienced, when does this occur (day or night)?

24. Does the person appear tired during or after eating?

25. Are there certain foods the person seems unable to tolerate?

26. What (if anything) does the person eat most?

With the answers to as many of these questions as possible, it becomes easier for the physician or practitioner to understand what is required to ease the situation. People can develop allergies or intolerances for certain food groups. Keeping a food diary can provide another helpful record.

Physical issues such as difficulty in swallowing can feel alarming and put people off eating. Sometimes less mucus is produced, so the mouth and throat get very dry, which makes swallowing difficult. Ensure that people have access to fluids and softer foods.

Some people find chewing difficult. Tooth pain, ill-fitting dentures or a sore mouth will impact negatively, so ensure regular oral checkups. Provide opportunities for people to swill their mouths (and spit out!).

Bouts of coughing or choking can lead to the person inhaling particles of food or liquid into their lungs, which is extremely uncomfortable. This has the potential to lead to bacterial infection, causing pneumonia (aspiration pneumonia). This can be treated with antibiotics, but it is far better to avoid these problems. Coughing and choking can be caused by stress, dryness of the throat, reflux/phlegm issues, blockages, drowsiness and decreased muscle movement.

Make the eating environment as inviting as possible. Keep mealtimes relaxed. This is a huge challenge in many care settings, as it is one of the most anxious and stressful times of the day. Lots of people are on the move and there is often a limited time-frame or a set routine. It may be easier to create a more relaxed environment over mealtimes at home.

Anxiety can increase the sensation of choking. This is partly because anxiety increases our sensitivity to regular bodily functions, and we become more aware of the experience of swallowing than most people. This heightened awareness changes the act of swallowing from an unconscious action to something that feels more deliberate and awkward.

People sometimes feel as though they have a lump in their throat obstructing the passage of food, and we have seen this sensation disappear when the person feels more relaxed. However, it is also important to get things checked out to alleviate anxieties or deal with any physical problems. Depression is also known to suppress appetite.

Indigestion, heartburn and reflux are very common and often painful conditions experienced in older age. When we swallow food, it passes down the oesophagus through a valve into the stomach. However, stomach acid can leak back through the valve causing pain in the chest and a bitter taste in the mouth. People living with dementia, particularly in later stages, may be unable to say where they are experiencing pain. They may wake in the night, or be restless, wanting to get up because the acid reflux is so uncomfortable.

If the person is uncomfortable at night, try raising the head end of the bed about six inches. It is not always helpful to use lots of pillows for a semi-sitting position, because this tends to put pressure on the stomach. Better to raise the legs of the bed at the head end, so that the body can lie at a slight angle. Some people state that sleeping on their left side is helpful too.

Less acidic foods may help to relieve the problem: oatmeal, melon, banana; grilled, steamed or baked chicken or fish; green vegetables, carrots and potatoes. Not eating for three hours before going to bed will also help. This gives the food time to be digested and pass beyond where it is likely to cause regurgitation or acid reflux.

Difficulty in chewing or swallowing can also be alleviated through the use of blended food. Many healthy people are using blended foods and smoothies as part of their fitness regime, so there is less stigma attached to needing to eat minced meals. The food can still be shaped and presented well; brightened with a sprig of parsley or flavoured with herbs and spices.

Food

MAKE YOUR OWN SMOOTHIE RECIPE

Fruit and vegetable smoothies can be delicious. List fruits and flavours that the person enjoys. Use it to help choose the main ingredients for a new smoothie. Blend ingredients for one to two minutes until smooth, and serve immediately. Some people like to drink directly from the cup. Others prefer to use a spoon. Here are two smoothie recipes we enjoyed making.

GREEN SMOOTHIE

Blend the following ingredients:

I apple, peeled and chopped

I avocado, peeled and chopped

(Optional) I celery stick, chopped

2 cups of steamed spinach or kale

2 cups of apple juice

FRUIT SMOOTHIE

Blend the following ingredients:

I banana

½ tin of apricots

¼ cup of juice (apple, orange or apricot)

½ cup of soya milk or yogurt

FOOD FOR THOUGHT

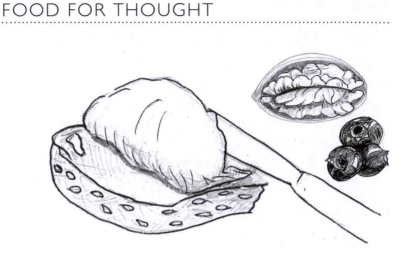

Figure 4.5: Mackerel pâté, mix flaked smoked mackerel, crème fraîche, lemon juice and a good dash of horseradish, walnuts and blueberries

Anything that is good for the body, such as fresh fruit and vegetables, grains, seeds, proteins, nuts, etc., is good for the brain. Many people like the idea of superfoods that are full of vitamins and antioxidants (nutrients that prevent cell damage). There are mixed opinions about how super these foods are, but blueberries and avocado feature regularly in talks about healthy foods.

Omega 3 fats are also good for healthy brain function. They are found in mackerel, tuna, pilchards, kippers, salmon and herring, soya bean oil, linseed oil, pumpkin seeds and walnuts.

'Food for Thought' is an event with a healthy food buffet and a thought-provoking question or statement about any subject. This type of session has often stimulated conversations that surprise people, as though we were immediately reaping the benefits of healthy foods!

There are some important statements to put in place first. Write these out and read them aloud to ensure everyone has the opportunity to know that:

1. There are no right or wrong answers. People have different opinions.
2. Some thoughts take a long time to formulate.
3. There is no rush or pressure to contribute today.

Use any theme that may be of interest to the person/people you are with. Sample thought cards might be:

○ Why are we here? What is the meaning of human life?

○ Is there life somewhere else in the universe?

○ Home is where the heart is.

○ 'Food comes first, and then morality.' (Bertolt Brecht)

PICNIC

Picnics feel special and exciting at any time of year. There is a sense of liberation about eating outside. Most of our day trips to a park, a beach, or woodlands involve a picnic with a view. Getting fresh air can build an appetite and there is great satisfaction in eating whilst noticing the scenery or wildlife. People love trying to get the birds closer to the picnic spread.

Preparations for the picnic can be a shared family/group activity. Have images or names of places to choose from. Make the sandwiches or bake together. Picnic preparation increases the anticipation of a good day. Pack the plates, cutlery. Small pots or jars can be used for seasoning and sauces. It is easy to take bottled water and juices. Take a small cutting board and one sharp knife, kept in a container, for cutting fruit or cheese.

Moist hand wipes and kitchen wipes or towels for accidental spills are useful; also a bag for rubbish. Take picnic blankets, even if sitting on benches or camping chairs, as they are useful for cushions or for wrapping around cold knees. Plastic bags or bin liners can be useful to spread over wet benches. Ensure that all plastics and rubbish are collected before you leave the area.

Rarely is this a major issue, but occasionally we are visited by stinging and biting insects. These pesky creatures can be deterred by wrapping up well and applying effective lotions such as *Avon Bug Guard*, *Smidge Spray*, *Bushman's Repellant*, *Shoo*, or home-made citronella, olive oil and Dettol mixes. Avoid bananas, as it seems they attract insects. Have anti-histamine cream or calamine lotion ready to dab on bites to reduce the irritating itch.

Take photographs of the picnic, the place, and the people. These photographs can later stimulate conversation about the day, or be presented as an option for future days out.

HIGH TEA

Another exciting and social event is high tea, of which there are two versions. High tea or, as it was known, 'afternoon tea' became popular in the early nineteenth century. It was mostly the activity of upper class people who had tea with sandwiches and cakes whilst seated in armchairs, between 4.00 pm and 6.00 pm, before the main dinner.

Less wealthy families had high tea on Sundays, comprising sandwiches, cold meats and pastries. In industrialised working-class places, high tea was the evening meal taken at the kitchen table when the workers came home. They needed good hot food rather than sandwiches and cakes.

Today high tea is regarded as a treat that many hotels offer. But it is such fun to create an old-fashioned version of high tea at home or in a care setting. Create decorative place cards. Make dainty crackers by rolling pretty wrapping paper around a rolled up piece of paper containing a note about etiquette or an interesting piece of information. Tie them with ribbons and place one on each person's plate.

Use beautiful napkins. Dress up for the occasion. Many charity shops or second-hand stores sell vintage clothes – or just a hat or a pair of gloves will be transformative. Make a fan. Put flowers on the table. Such events create an atmosphere of joyfulness. Many are the times we have watched people's body posture lengthen and straighten as they play their part in the high tea.

SKETCHING MOVEMENT

This activity involves half the people moving, while the other half create quick sketches of the movement. Then they swap places, so everyone has an opportunity to be the person moving, and the artist capturing the movement.

You could look at draft movement sketches by French artist Edgar Degas. He is known for his paintings capturing the movement of ballet dancers and horses. He did quick sketches while at the ballet, but completed his paintings in the studio. The art we create may be of a different standard to Degas, but it can still be fun and effective. Again, we make it clear that there is no right or wrong way to move or sketch.

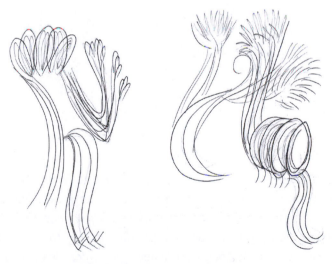

Figure 4.6: A movement sketch

Begin with a gentle warm-up for everyone. This starts with the breathing exercise and then asks people to wriggle their fingers. Extend that movement into their wrists: gently turning their wrists leads to their arms moving, at first close to the bodies, but gradually extending, using elbow and shoulder movements. Stop if there is any sign of discomfort. Keep the movements soft and fluid.

Next, do some music doodles to relax people into the experience of moving to music and conveying the movement in space with movements on paper, using colour pens, pastels or crayons. This can be done seated at the table, or standing with paper on clip-boards – whatever feels best.

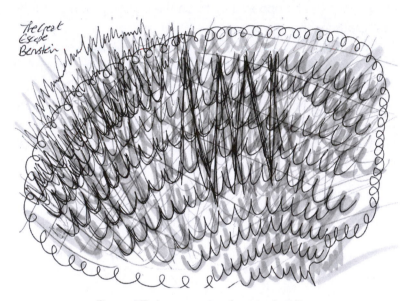

Figure 4.7: An example of music doodling:
The Great Escape by Elmer Bernstein

The artists are given fresh paper and asked to write their name in the corner. The dancers or movers begin to move. The artists' job is to capture the movement they see. They need to focus on the movement and not on the person making the movement. This concept can be tricky, but a few music doodles and a quick demonstration will help establish the aims of this activity.

The movers or dancers may be seated or standing. Their job is to move in whatever way they can to music. Use classical or pop music. If people are fit, they might dance for a whole five to ten minutes, which gives a good amount of time for sketching detailed movement.

If people feel less energised, try a staggered routine. This is where each dancer moves for 15 to 30 seconds before the next dancer takes over. Initially people may feel embarrassed, so 15 seconds is easier to manage. Highlight the importance of the artists creating lines of movement, and that we may not see any actual bodies in the sketches, just the outlines of a swoosh, or a high arm, or a bent head.

Allow a couple of minutes after the movement has stopped for the artists to complete any of the lines they have started. Then swap over the roles.

After everyone has had an opportunity to sketch and move, either ask people to show their images and describe the experience, or place the images together on the floor and look for patterns or similarities. Quite often the images are stunningly unique.

Sleep

Sleep enables the body and mind to relax and recuperate. It is essential for physical health and healthy brain function. Sleep helps the body maintain the right hormone levels; it helps keep the immune system healthy, and enables cells to repair.

Lack of sleep is very stressful and can cause damage and imbalance to our blood sugar levels, weight, and ability to cope with life. Sleep deprivation affects our moods and our ability to think clearly. Things can feel out of proportion, which in turn increases our anxiety levels.

In dementia care, there may be several possible causes for sleeping problems. Rose, Fagin and Lorenz (2010)[13] note that disturbance of the brain's wake/sleep cycle can be caused by neurological damage and various medications. Lack of quality sleep leads to daytime napping, which can cause further night sleep problems. Increased daytime activity and daylight are known to help people sleep better.

A short 20-minute sleep is unlikely to cause night problems. Relaxation and rest can help rejuvenate the body. But longer naps in the daytime can affect the quality and length of sleep at night. People sometimes take naps to ease pain or boredom, or so that the carer can have a much needed break. Some people sleep during the day because there is 'nothing to be awake for'.

Use the various activities to help stimulate people with gentle exercise, fresh air and friendly company. Good sleeps of around seven to eight hours at night help the body repair and recover.

References

1. Martin, L.R., Williams, S.L., Haskard, K.B. and DiMatteo, M.R. (2005) 'The challenge of patient adherence.' *Therapeutics and Clinical Risk Management 1*, 3, 189–199. www.ncbi.nlm.nih.gov/pmc/articles/PMC 1661624. Accessed on 30 June 2015.

2. Hall, J.A., Roter, D.L., Milburn, M.A. and Daltroy, L.H. (1996) 'Patients' health as a predictor of physician and patient behavior in medical visits: A synthesis of four studies.' *Medical Care 34*, 12, 1205–18.

3. Hoffman S.J. (2013) 'Following celebrities' medical advice: Meta-narrative analysis.' *British Medical Journal 347*. Available at www.bmj.com/content/347/bmj.f7151. Accessed on 30 June 2015.

4. Nicolai, S., Benzinger, P., Skelton, D.A., Aminian, K., Becker, C. and Lindemann, U. (2010) 'Day-to-day variability of physical activity of older adults living in the community.' *Journal of Aging and Physical Activity 18*, 75–86.

5. Henson, J., Yates T., Biddle, S.J., Edwardson, C.L., Khunti, K., Wilmot E.G. *et al.* (2013) 'Associations of objectively measured sedentary behaviour and physical activity with markers of cardiometabolic health.' *Diabetologia 56*, 5,1012–20. doi: 10.1007/s00125-013-2845-9. Epub 1 March 2013. Available at www.ncbi.nlm.nih.gov/pubmed/23456209. Accessed on 5 July 2015. See also: Wilmot, E.G.I., Edwardson, C.L., Achana, F.A., Davies, M.J., Gorely, T., Gray, L.J. *et al.* (2012) 'Sedentary time in adults and the association with diabetes, cardiovascular disease and death: Systematic review and meta-analysis.' *Diabetologia 55*, 11, 2895–905. doi: 10.1007/s00125-012-2677-z. Epub 14 August 2012.

6. DoH (2011) *Start Active, Stay Active: A Report On Physical Activity for Health From the Four Home Countries' Chief Medical Officers.* London: Department of Health.

7. WHO (2011) *Global Recommendations on Physical Activity for Health.* Available at www.who.int/dietphysicalactivity/factsheet_recommendations /en. Accessed on 14 August 2015.

8. Alzheimer Australia NSW (2014) *The Benefits of Physical Activity and Exercise for People Living with Dementia.* Discussion Paper 11, November 2014. Available at nsw.fightdementia.org.au/sites/default/files/NSW/documents/AANSW_DiscussionPaper11.pdf. Accessed on 14 August 2015. (This paper has been developed by the Policy, Research and Information Department, Alzheimer's Australia NSW. Paper authored by Kylie Miskovski, Senior Research and Policy Officer, Alzheimer's Australia NSW.)

9. Goldsworthy, A. (1990) *A Collaboration With Nature.* New York: Abrams.

10. Goldsworthy, A. (2011) *Stone.* London: Thames & Hudson.

11. Sagan C. (1985) Contact. London: Orbit.

12. Longfellow, H. W. 'Evangeline: A Tale of Arcadie.' In L. Buell (ed) (1988) *Selected Poems.* London: Penguin Books.

13. Rose, K. M., Fagin, C. M. and Lorenz, R. (2010). 'Sleep disturbances in dementia: What they are and what to do.' *Journal of Gerontological Nursing* 36, 5, 9–14. doi:10.3928/00989134-20100330-05. Available at www.ncbi.nlm.nih.gov/pmc/articles/PMC3062259. Accessed on 14 August 2014.

5

SUPPORTING SELF-EXPRESSION

We are creative beings. We recognise and respond to expressions of creativity, be they beautiful landscaped gardens; delicious lemon drizzle cake; a child's first painting; a love poem; furniture designs; patterns in the pavement; a film; music; dance; the shape of a vase; or the colours and textures of textiles. It is in our nature to express ourselves through creativity.

Self-expression is the communication of our stories, feelings, thoughts, or ideas. We may express our individuality through what we say and how we say it, or through the clothes and colours that we wear. Self-expression is a sharing of who we are, our life experiences, spirit, passions or knowledge. People use a variety of art forms to convey their authentic selves.

The freedom of expression is a human right that applies to everyone, including people in the latter stages of dementia. Article 10 of the Human Rights Act 1998 states people have the right of freedom to communicate and express themselves in any medium, including words, actions and images. Artistic expression is strongly protected.

Self-expression is an important aspect of integrity. People diagnosed with dementia may feel disconnection and loss, but through expression of these feelings they can feel an integration of different parts of themselves. This sense of wholeness and meaning promotes mental wellbeing.

We are narrative beings and have stories about moments in time that help validate our identity, especially when heard and valued. But many people living with brain disease or other long-term conditions experience fewer opportunities to be heard. If verbal communication is difficult, chances for positive self-expression are narrower.

> Not only do we exist in a story-telling world but our very Selves are constituted by the stories we and others tell about ourselves… Some people find their stories marginalized, themselves as narrators dispossessed.
>
> (Baldwin 2008)[1]

When self-expression is blocked people can experience a loss of energy and power, or a great sense of anger and frustration. These emotions may show up as depression and be expressed in ways that either feel negative or lead to undesirable outcomes. This is the experience of people whose label of dementia renders them deficient, impaired or incapable. But it is not OK for anyone to be silenced through stigma and discrimination.

Williams and Keady (2006)[2] confirm that the concept of narrative approaches to dementia care is well established, and yet still sometimes misses the voices of people living with dementia. This may partly be due to people's lack of confidence in inspiring narrative expression.

In Ward, Cambell and Keady's (2014)[3] beautiful exploration of the meaning of appearance to people living with dementia, we find rich narratives when expression is supported. The colours and clothes people chose (or would have chosen if permitted) had personal meaning and direct links to a parent, or personal or community memory. One gentleman's attention to shaving and wearing a tie was in relation to his father, and an honouring of standards that were part of his identity. The work shows the importance of appearance for self-expression.

> I want freedom for the full expression of my personality.
>
> (Mahatma Gandhi)

People living with dementia can connect and express themselves through creativity, without exception. It is our role to create and share expressive opportunities. This requires families and care staff to tap into their own creativity and that means letting go of limiting personal beliefs.

Narrative work does not have to be in words. People tell stories through art, painting, musical expression, singing, dance and movement. The narrative moment does not have to be in the past. It can be here and now, in this shared moment. The story does not have to be fully understood. Some of the best stories are glimpses into a mysterious narrative such as:

'And then he kissed me. Love is a good thing.'

'He's had a shock, but he can still sing like Elvis.'

Nind (2008)[4] shows a variety of ways to conduct research with people with learning, communication and other disabilities. These methods offer perfectly relevant guidance for supporting self-expression and narrative work. She also quotes Aldridge (2007),[5] who used participatory photographic methods so that people with a learning disability could express their views through the images they chose to capture. This means the focus is on what people can do, rather than on their incapacity.

Therein lies one of the fundamental principles in positive dementia care: our recognition and focus need to be on capability, even when disease is causing cognitive difficulties. People still have capacity for self-expression and connection. Most of the activities below have engaged people whose relatives or care staff had not believed engagement was possible. They had been caught up in the story of loss and decline that is assumed to be synonymous with the label 'dementia'.

Atkinson (2004)[6] has used qualitative research, oral history and life-story work with people with learning difficulties, in ways that value and validate people's individual accounts. The process has helped many people tell their stories and 'challenge people and events in their lives, denounce practices and provide alternative social histories'. The activities to support identity in Chapter 1 have been used in dementia care, as well as to support people to express sensitive issues (Marshall and Tilley 2013).[7]

Cultural differences in self-expression

Kim and Markus (2002)[8] noted that thoughts are regularly verbalised in western culture to the extent that some people find it difficult to solve problems or function without speaking aloud. Speech is the primary means of self-expression.

However, in East Asian cultures thoughtful silence is often valued more highly than speech.

Self-expression is not commonly encouraged. Instead, as noted by Tobin (2005),[9] the emphasis is on intuiting feelings more than expressing feelings. From an early age, children are taught to be empathic and anticipate the needs of others. Empathy in Japan means being aware of the non-verbalised feelings of other people. (This is known as advanced empathy in the UK.) Emotions are expressed, but in the 'right way' at the 'right time' – modified to fit the context. This concept appears in western culture manners too, but is less strongly emphasised. In Australia, America and Western Europe there is a preference for people to 'always be themselves' under any and all conditions. That includes being free to express themselves. The concept of freedom of expression as a human right is only around 70 years old in Japan, in comparison to a human rights history spanning 800 years in the UK.

Being aware of cultural differences is useful in dementia care, partly for the obvious purpose of supporting people with different cultural backgrounds, but also because it raises our awareness about diverse perspectives on issues that we have assumed are of universal importance.

There are differences between collectivism and individualism in behaviour, values and attitudes. Collectivism tends to place greater importance on harmony with others: fitting in and fulfilling social obligations. But in an era of expanding communication, travel and cross-cultural integration there will be a range of experiences.

Stephan *et al.* (1998)[10] does not believe that collectivism and individualism are opposite ends of one spectrum. His research shows individualism and collectivism to be 'a loose collection of many cultural characteristics', some of which are consistent, and some of which are not consistent with expected displays of emotion and self-expression. Nothing can be assumed. What matters is providing opportunities, again and again, for individuals to express their personal and/or cultural selves.

Offering the best opportunity

Over the years I have developed the following tips towards successful outcomes for creative expression in dementia care.

- Make things accessible: physically people may need things adjusting (chair height; arm rests on chairs; table height). Visually, people need good light and the materials need to be clearly visible.

- Always remember you are working with an adult. The person with dementia has a lifetime of experience that still exists and is worthy of respect, regardless of ability to communicate.

- Use colour contrasts: work on a plain coloured surface. People struggle to see things on a patterned background.

- Make things achievable: do not set people up to fail, but at the same time ensure work is interesting and relevant to the person. Focus on the benefits of the process rather than the outcome. Break every task down into achievable steps.

- Allow control over the task: regard the person you are with as an artist in their own right. What they choose to do on the page is their business. Ask them to choose colours or patterns they like. Ensure there are choices.

- Expectation without pressure... This is a way of being that makes a huge difference to the quality of the experience. Expect people to be able to do the activity. Expect people to engage and enjoy themselves. Expect that you have the skills and ability to facilitate the process. Expect the activity to show what works well and what could be different. Expect connection...and then find a way to do the work without putting pressure on anybody to 'perform'. (With practice this approach gets better and better at supporting people to express their creativity.)

Every child is an artist. The problem is how to remain an artist once he grows up.

(Pablo Picasso)

ACTIVITIES TO SUPPORT SELF EXPRESSION

Cameron (1995)[11] suggests setting aside blocks of time (called an 'artist's date') purely for nurturing our inner creative beings. This could be taking two hours a week to inspire our artistic selves by exploring places we have seen; going to a play; looking through secondhand clothing stores; visiting an aquarium, a model railway shop, a haberdashery or art gallery. Sometimes the 'artist's date' might be to sit and look through beautiful books or magazines or sort through the old art materials box.

Most of the following activities are designed to be done by individuals within a group or in pairs.

MUSIC DOODLES

'Music doodles' (or 'scribbles') is one of the most easily accessible creative activities for promoting unhindered self-expression. Used in care and community settings with people living with all stages of dementia, this pastime really lifts the spirits. I include it in every learning programme and even use it whilst writing.

Music accompanies our lives from cradle to grave. There is a song, chant, hymn or piece of music for every occasion. Most of us, living with or without dementia, can make a connection to and through music. Whether or not we can play an instrument, we have the capacity to imagine playing or conducting the music we hear.

Listening to music appears to improve our mood and can increase memory function, attention span and language abilities (Särkämo et al. 2008; Jäncke 2009).[12,13] Playing music is even better!

In their review of ways in which music and singing relate to health and wellbeing, Stacy, Brittain and Kerr (2002)[14] affirm that music can induce relaxation and have physical, emotional, spiritual and social benefits.

'Music doodles' requires some paper and colour markers (felt pens or preferably oil pastels), and some loud classical music. Use a board to support the paper if the person is in bed; otherwise do the activity at the table. The only instruction is to allow the music to guide the hand around the page, using whichever colours the person prefers. There is no need to draw anything that resembles anything else. There is no right or wrong interpretation of the music, just a sense of flowing with the sounds.

We use the following pieces of music:

○ Strauss's 'Blue Danube'

○ Mozart's *'Eine Kleine Nachtmusik'* (allegro)

○ Bernstein's 'The Great Escape'.

The fuller orchestral sound offers more opportunities for people to latch on to a particular sound, rhythm or instrument. Most results show unique scribbles, although 'The Great Escape' tends to show similar markings, because the beat is so strong throughout the piece. Offer to play the piece a second time and swap colours. Often people take most of the first play to relax into the activity, so the second time around feels better.

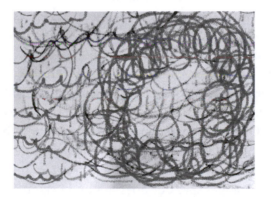

Figure 5.1: Example of a music doodle (Strauss)

The doodles may show circles and swirls from the sound of violins, or individual marks of single notes. The outcome is not as important as the process of self-expression through the music. Use a cardboard frame to see how different parts of the image appear. Some can be surprisingly beautiful…and all are unique!

Sounds and voice warm-ups

Some people living with intermediate and late stages of dementia tell us that they don't use their voices much, or that their voices are weak. Regularly, people speak less when they find that their meaning is not being understood or their words are confused. They refer others to their partner or carer to answer questions on their behalf.

If the voice is underused the muscles around the vocal folds may weaken. This can lead to whispery or hoarse sound quality, making conversation difficult. People may need more breath to be able to speak. This is partly because the weakened muscles have more gaps and let air escape. The voice warm-up activity will help strengthen vocal chords over a three-week period.

Voices are valuable means of self-expression. By an announcement or a scream, for example, we let people know how we feel and what we want. If someone experiences less control over their life circumstances and choices, being heard takes on greater significance.

We can support people in their communication by allowing time for them to find words. Jumping in with our own words is neither helpful nor desirable for someone trying to express him- or herself. Our role is to support self-expression. This requires trusting in the ability of the person to communicate. Carers may struggle to believe this is possible. Often carers say the person they support cannot speak or does not understand anything; but through creative interaction they discover that the person can and does.

Noise levels in the environment affect how well a person hears. Difficulties in speech comprehension in older adults are often put down to cognitive decline. Daneman (2005)[15] notes that one of the prevalent theories links lack of speech comprehension with a generalised slowing down of brain function with age. But sensory decline (hearing impairment) may well be the cause. So check hearing levels and hearing aids.

Occasionally people choose not to speak as a way of preserving themselves. This is known in mental health care and care in long-stay institutions. The choice of using the voice, or being silent, is also one of the few things people may have control over.

WARMING UP THE VOICE (1)

The warm-up activity offers a way of using the voice without any pressure to speak or converse. We use it in a variety of settings and love the way people who are not known to speak, feel able to join in. It is vital that the person does not feel pressured into speaking. The purpose of this and every activity is to have fun and make a connection. Follow the directions here as a basic framework.

1. Begin with noticing our breathing and gently slow it down. No need for huge breaths. Just keep it gentle and slow.
2. Take a breath and hum any note for any length of time. With two or more people, hum in turns to keep the sound going. After a few rounds, people find a rhythm that makes the breathing and the humming easy to maintain. There is no obligation to get this 'right' on any occasion.
3. Now try the following sounds. The 'Eeee' sound often resonates and can sound very beautiful, even with just two voices. There is no set note – just experiment with high-pitch and low-pitch sounds.
   a. Eeeee
   b. Ahhhh
   c. Ooooo
   d. Eeeee

WARMING UP THE VOICE (2)

The next warm-up is to loosen the lips and give the vocal chords a rest.

Try vibrating your lips as you blow out through your mouth with your lips closed. This could sound like a contented horse. Now add vocal sound to the lip vibrations by going up and down a musical scale. This is often very funny as people splutter to keep the sounds going.

Now use more vocal sounds with a musical scale such as:

'Ma mi mo ma mi mo ma mi'

'La li lo la li lo la li'

'Do ray me far so la te do'

Finish the warm-ups with the 'Eeee' sound and notice how much longer the note can be sustained, and how much it resonates. If working with a group, suggest that people create their own sound for others to follow. Create sounds for how people feel at this moment in time. These could range from big sighs to a shrill trill, as if in celebration.

SONG WRITING

Singer-songwriters have been expressing aspects of their life for many years. Lyrics by recording artists such as Johnny Cash, Bob Dylan, Joan Baez, Joni Mitchell, Van Morrison, Leonard Cohen, Annie Lennox, Kate Bush and Bjork express songs about love, loss and personal experiences.

Begin with examples of different types of songs and explore which ones people enjoy most.

○ Ballads – songs that tell a story from beginning to end (sometimes with a chorus).

○ Folk – another type of story-song that may refer to social or political issues.

○ Jazz – African/American and American origins – also uses improvisation, so the song may change each time it is sung.

- Gospel – uses strong vocal harmonies and is often in praise of God or celebrating God's love.

- Country – the lyrics are the main part of country songs and may convey a personal incident in great detail.

- Rap – is like thinking out loud, sharing who you are, to a clear rhythm.

- Pop – pop (popular) songs came out of rock 'n' roll in the 1950s and are usually verse–chorus–verse–chorus–structure, short or medium songs with catchy tunes.

COMPOSING A SONG

A simple way to create a song is to take a theme and list as many words as possible linked to that theme. If there are no musicians around, use a tune that people are generally familiar with and create the new lyrics using the list of words. Work around a theme, such as:

- Breakfasts I have enjoyed.

- The day I fell in love.

- My heart is like…

- My memory is…

Approach everything with a 'try it and see' attitude. Here was an attempt at a 'Breakfast song' to the tune of 'Twinkle, twinkle, little star':

> 'Breakfast comes before the post
> Scrambled or fried eggs on toast
> Bacon, mushrooms and brown sauce
> With a cup of tea of course
> Now it's time for buttered toast
> With marmalade I love the most.

Most songs are made up of verses and choruses. The words are different for each verse and convey the meaning of the song (the story, message or emotion). The chorus is usually the catchy bit that is repeated throughout the song. It can be fun to try variations on a theme. You can use any sentence or phrase that is already around you. This gives the song some personal meaning. Offer pens and paper with a list of words that need to be rhymed with.

'My memory is like a dolphin' contained phrases people used to describe their dementia:

> My memory's like a dolphin
> It comes and goes
> Like the sea it ebbs and flows
> Like a sieve I can see through the holes.
>
>> To the bright stars in the sky
>> That shine on invisible
>> We're made of stars in the night
>> We shine on invincible.
>
> And I'm feeling good inside my soul
> It's where I want to meet you (yeah)
> So hold my hand and understand
> That we're doing fine, on this unknown journey.
>
>> To the bright stars in the sky
>> That shine on invisible
>> We're made of stars in the night
>> We shine on invincible.

PAINTING IN THE STYLE OF...

If you do not know where to start with creative expression, look at images by those who have successfully expressed themselves: Picasso, Van Gogh, Miro, Matisse and more contemporary artists such as Hopper, Hockney, Emin and Perry. We find that people from a wide variety of cultures, with and without dementia, can appreciate art and the stories behind the artists.

Focus on three or four artists in a year. Explore their history and different styles of painting. If possible visit art galleries, take an art tour, study library books. Try a short online arts history course. Immerse yourself in the world of the great artists. Some art galleries offer guided tours or dementia-friendly talks.

You could start by copying the styles of other artists. This is how Constable learned to paint so well! One of the more relaxing and popular activities is to emulate the swirls in Van Gogh's 'Starry night' across the page, using thick paint to get texture and movement. Even if it looks a complete mess, it feels great!

Some people with dementia really enjoy painting in the style of Piet Mondrian, who was able to take a complex image and paint it in its simplest form. Artists Piet Mondrian and Hans Hoffman painted beautiful and detailed images of nature, but they also painted the essence of things, using blocks of colour. In our experience people with dementia are moving further towards this way of interpreting the world…describing the essence of objects, being the essence of human-beingness.

Look at an area of the room you are in and see whether you can represent it in blocks of colour, rather than by realistic lines and shapes. The outcomes can be extremely effective modern pieces of art.

Another favourite artist is Henri Matisse, particularly in his cut-out phase towards the end of his life when he was unwell. Matisse cut shapes out of coloured paper to arrange in ways that are vivid and memorable. This style of art is accessible and offers results quite quickly. You could experiment by cutting one shape and gluing it to a shape of a different colour, to layer the art.

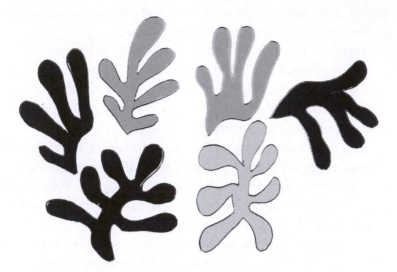

Figure 5.2: Matisse-style paper cut-outs

I Remember Better When I Paint (2009) is a film by Berna Huebner who explored her mother's journey through Alzheimer's disease. The film is narrated by Olivia de Havilland, presented by the Hilgos Foundation and French Connection Films. The film has been shown worldwide. It is a moving testimony to the power of painting for quality of life. For more information visit https://irememberbetterwhenipaint.wordpress.com.

CLAY WORK

Working with clay just feels good! Use air-drying clay for ease. You will also need some water, a plastic knife and optional plastic gloves and aprons, plus plastic wrapping to keep unused clay fresh.

You can make anything you want, or just experience the feel of the clay.

SCULPT A DOG OUT OF CLAY

For an accessible and effective result try the following activity to make a dog lying down:

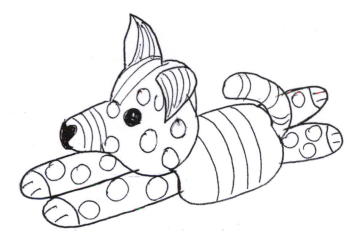

Figure 5.3: Clay dog

1. Make two sausage shapes and lay them side-by-side. The ends of the sausages will become the front and back legs.
2. Make an oval shape to place on top of the sausage shapes in the middle, for the body. Score some marks into the clay with the knife and add some water to help the body stick to the legs.
3. Smooth the body edges over the sides of legs so that it all sticks together.
4. Make a ball shape for the head and pull one part into a snout. Place it firmly on the front of the body, above the front legs. Use the knife to score marks in the clay to help it stick.
5. Stretch up two points on the head to make ears.

6. Add a tiny ball (or a bead) for the nose.

7. Finally, roll a thinner piece of clay to form the tail and stick it onto your dog's body.

8. When the clay is properly dry (allow 24 hours) you can paint it.

Hold an exhibition of your self-expressive art!

References

1. Baldwin, C. (2008) 'Narrative, citizenship and dementia: The personal and the political.' *Journal of Aging Studies, 22*, 222–228.

2. Williams, J. and Keady, J. (2006) Editorial: 'The narrative voice of people with dementia.' *Dementia: The International Journal of Research and Practice 5*, 2,163–166.

3. Ward, R., Campbell, S. and Keady, J. (2014) 'Once I had money in my pocket, I was every colour under the sun': Using "appearance biographies" to explore the meanings of appearance for people with dementia.' *Journal of Aging Studies 30*, 64–72. Available at www.sciencedirect.com/science/article/pii/S0890406514000280. Accessed on 6 July 2015.

4. Nind, M. (2008) 'Conducting qualitative research with people with learning, communication and other disabilities: Methodological challenges.' ESRC National Centre for Research Methods Review Paper. Southampton: National Centre for Research Methods, University of Southampton.

5. Aldridge, J. (2007) 'Picture this: The use of participatory photographic research methods with people with learning disabilities.' *Disability and Society 22*, 1, 1–17.

6. Atkinson, D. (2004) 'Research and empowerment: Involving people with learning difficulties in oral and life history research.' *Disability and Society 19*, 7, 961–702.

7. Marshall, K. and Tilley, E. (2013) 'Life stories, intellectual disability, cultural heritage and ethics: Dilemmas in researching and (re)presenting accounts from the Scottish Highlands.' *Ethics and Social Welfare 7*, 3, 400–409.

8. Kim, H.S. and Markus, H.R. (2002). 'Freedom of Speech and Freedom of Silence: An Analysis of Talking as a Cultural Practice.' In R. Shweder, M. Minow and H. R. Markus (eds) *Engaging Cultural Differences: The Multicultural Challenge in Liberal Democracies*. New York: Russell-Sage Foundation.

9. Tobin J. (2005) 'The irony of self-expression.' *American Journal of Education 103*, 3, 233–258. Available at www.joetobin.net/pdf/Jtobin-IronyofSelfExpression.pdf. Accessed on 14 August 2015.

10. Stephan, C.W., Stephan, W.G., Saito, I. and Barnett, S.M. (1998) 'Emotional expression in Japan and the United States: The non-monolithic nature of individualism and collectivism.' *Journal of Cross-Cultural Psychology 29*, 6, 728–748.
11. Cameron, J. (1995) *The Artist's Way*. London: Pan Macmillan.
12. Särkämö, T., Tervaniemi, M., Laitinen, S., Forsblom, A., Soinila, S., Mikkonen, M. *et al.* (2008) 'Music listening enhances cognitive recovery and mood after middle cerebral artery stroke.' *Brain 131*, 866–876. doi: 10.1093/brain/awn013.
13. Jäncke, L. (2009) 'Music drives brain plasticity.' *F1000 Reports Biology 1*, 78. doi: 10.3410/BI78. Available at www.ncbi.nlm.nih.gov/pmc/articles/PMC2948283 Accessed 10 October 2015.
14. Stacy, R., Brittain, K. and Kerr, S. (2002) 'Singing for Health: An exploration of the issues.' *Health Education 102*, 4, 156–162.
15. Daneman, M. (2005) 'Speech comprehension difficulties in older adults: Cognitive slowing or age-related changes in hearing?' *Psychology and Aging 20*, 2, 261–271.

6

SUPPORT FOR WHEN A PERSON SEEMS CONFUSED

There seems to be a wisdom in people living with dementia that is deeper than many of us realise. It is only half heard, because it is not looked for. What we see in the person with dementia is confusion. We do not believe that it is we who are confused. Maybe we need to listen more, assume less…be alert to what may be evolving, because dementia is teaching us something.

Some families or care staff discover a connection beyond the sadness about the loss of cognitive abilities. It is a place of mindfulness and the essence of humanity. The journey to that place is rarely direct and often difficult. Maybe it could be easier if people tuned into the wisdom earlier. But we are very used to focusing on what everyone else highlights, and what we focus on increases.

Confusion is, however, a natural state. It may feel uncomfortable, but when we allow it, confusion can lead us to learn far more, and be clearer about what is important. Confusion is the feeling of bewilderment and uncertainty about something. When faced with a new problem or dilemma we feel unclear about the way forward. But that does not mean something is wrong.

Confusion can help us find deeper wisdom as we search around for solutions. But often we are under time pressure to find clarity immediately. Pressure can make the situation worse and set people up to make a decision they were not ready for. Allow time to be with the confusion. Understand that confusion is natural and part of the bigger process. It can yield great results.

Kapura and Bielaczyca (2012)[1] explored confusion and learning in maths students. The students who had no initial instruction explored many approaches with uncertainty, trying to answer complex mathematical problems. They failed do so. Students who received direct instruction from the beginning found successful solutions. But the surprise is that when the first students did receive instruction they scored higher results in the post-test than those who had received instruction from the beginning. This suggests that their confusion and searching had opened their minds to be able to receive the information they really needed. Please remember this point.

In its mildest form most of us have expressed feelings of confusion about what day it is, or been muddled about a conversation topic. Given a little time, we are able to get back on track. There are, of course, more acute forms of confusion associated with dementia, intensified or caused by problems with memory, recognition, and the brain's ability to process information.

When phrases sound jumbled or confused, carers often think the person does not know what they are saying. However, it is our experience that the phrases often make perfect sense when we understand the context and references. Brain disease may be affecting language ability, but that does not mean the person is unaware of what they wish to communicate.

If we are familiar with the person's culture or context and have access to relevant images, we can move out of confusion to something understood. Confusion (our own, or other people's) needs the gift of time. It is interesting that when time is given for understanding and proper communication, less time is required to deal with the problems that arise when a person displays their unmet needs. The gift of time helps everybody.

The following are phrases that required time to understand:

- 'blue with the sheet' (image of the sea with a yacht)

- 'purple cold with balls on it' (purple cardigan with buttons)

- 'dingle dingle' (someone's at the door)

- 'the white that the queen sits on' (a baby's high chair).

It seems that the person is working hard to communicate by pulling out words that have some association with the missing word. Other words appear to have no relevance, but we can never really know, as we have not lived the same life. The word 'confusion' originates from the Latin for 'to pour together' or 'to mingle together'. It is an apt word for how it may feel to be unable to separate the desired word from all the others that exist.

If time is limited the carer can still acknowledge the person as a whole human being, simply by saying 'I know you are trying to tell me something. I'm having difficulty right now, but I want to understand you. Can we try again after I have...' This helps to value and validate the person.

Sometimes it is easier for strangers to do the valuing than for a relative who has grown tired of the confusion, and that is OK. Every person has days when they run out of patience, especially if the person being cared for is becoming abusive or upsetting to be with because of his or her own unmet needs. People need breaks from caring so that they can recharge and refocus on creating days that feel positive.

The feeling of confusion can be frightening. A person may be disorientated, not knowing where they are in terms of time, location and identity. Overstimulation can be a difficulty; too many voices or too many things going on. Large supermarket environments cause some people (both with and without dementia) to become overwhelmed by the vast array of information, noise, people and colours.

However, many shops and banks now display dementia-friendly signs (e.g. Alzheimer Scotland's blue flowers symbol indicating that the organisation is becoming dementia-friendly; or a knotted handkerchief sign, set up by Foton's Charity in the city of Bruges). These symbols help people know there are friendly staff who understand the need for quiet space.

In mid to later stages of dementia it can be useful to have a 'bag of tricks' like a Mary Poppins bag that contains everything you might ever need. This can really help to comfort, divert, distract, engage or calm a person who is becoming confused or upset. The bag can be taken on travel trips, visits or appointments. Each bag will be different to suit the individual, but as a general rule we have the following:

- snacks

- postcards, stamps, pen, address book

- images of spectacular buildings or natural beauty, or a magazine

- images of familiar people/places/things

- harmonica (mouth organ)

- lyrics to popular songs

- adult colouring-in pictures and felt pens

- a small travel blanket

- iPod and headphones

- personal communication book (see 'Activities').

Sometimes people find it difficult to make sense of things. The person may experience times of lucidity when neural pathways are flowing or can reroute, but at other times the most familiar things are unfathomable. If this confusion occurs it is important to slow everything down. Avoid using too many words. Allow more time. Offer calm and easy clues about what to do. Any rush or anxiety usually worsens the situation.

Research by Normann, Asplund and Norberg (1998)[2] found that people with severe dementia in care homes had spontaneous episodes of lucidity when working closely together with a carer who did not make demands on them, regarded them as valuable human beings, and saw their behaviours as meaningful expressions of their experiences.

If the person does not seem lucid, the carer needs to find a place of calmness (internally as much as externally) so that they can guide the person. Sometimes this is done in silence, giving visual clues or using body language to show the person what is needed. This ability to 'tune in' and value people is clearly important in dementia care.

It is worth checking possible reasons for increased states of confusion with a medical or dementia advisor. Causes may include:

- side effects of medication

- urinary tract infection

- being overheated

- sudden changes in brain function

- major life changes.

Use language that values people

Once a label is attached to someone, other people may take linguistic shortcuts to describe the way the person displays unmet needs. It is not acceptable to use language that diminishes the person, such as 'weeper', 'wanderer', 'sundowner' or 'attention seeker'.

Late afternoon changes

A person may experience changes around late afternoon, such as emotional anxiety or tension. This is sometimes referred to as 'sundowning'. Many of us experience a change in our mood as the daylight ends. For some this is a signal to get jobs finished and relax for the evening. For others it is a cause of unease. There are many possible reasons for changes. Here are a few suggestions and tips for helping someone feel more settled.

People may have been used to being busy in the late afternoon – making teas, driving home, preparing the children for bed, completing homework or reports, feeding the pets, cleaning, etc. Part of that busy feeling may still exist even when the person no longer does those jobs. This sense of anxiety that something should be happening can be distressing for people.

Tip: Prepare something meaningful to do around late afternoon, e.g. help prepare dinner/clean/sing/dance, or any other form of action.

The person may not be able to see clearly as the light fades. Dementia can affect eyesight, so semi-light appears much darker to some people.

Tip: Use brighter lights and have them switched on before the light fades, to reduce the change.

Dementia may cause disruption to the 24-hour body clock nerve cells, which can turn the whole wake/sleep pattern upside down. When we are winding down for the day, the person may be gearing up for the night.

Tip: One approach is to be physically active all day... Get walking, feed ducks, stretch, reduce daytime naps. This may help the person feel more ready to relax in the evenings.

If the person continues to be active during the night, ask if there are any care facilities that can support you. People need somewhere to go that is safe and active. In New York there is a night program for respite care. Care homes have the right facilities, so this much-needed service is likely to grow.

Walking

People use the term 'wandering' to describe people with dementia being on the move. The term usually implies that this activity is meaningless. That perspective is quite limiting. We may not know the purpose of their walking, but that does not make it worthless. Let us change the words and notice the difference in the way we view someone who walks as an adventurer, traveller, explorer, pioneer, pilgrim, commuter or voyager.

Why do we walk?

To see something new; get somewhere; move body and bowels; clear the mind; meet someone? People walk for a wide range of reasons. An ex-post office worker felt so much better when he walked with a bag to collect the mail from the front door and sort it into sizes and colours.

> For my dad, much of his walking was harking back to his life as a farmer and a gardener. Walking the fields, rounding up the cattle, sowing crops, ploughing and harvesting. Another man in the care home had also been a farmer, and if anything he walked even more than my dad. A female resident had very different reasons. She had been an executive and travelled extensively abroad for both business and pleasure, with a particular love of dancing the night away on cruise ships. Another lady had been a busy wife and mother all of her life,

and was used to being on her feet cleaning, tidying, cooking and running around after her children.

(Britton 2014)[3]

It is important to look beyond the label of dementia and be curious about the man or woman who walks the hallways.

Walking at night could be due to restless leg syndrome; needing the toilet; looking for a 'lost' partner; hunger; thirst; indigestion; or nightmares. Not everything is due to dementia. People communicate their unmet needs as best they can. Our work is to be curious and compassionate so that we can focus on the things that help.

A lot of our work with families and staff is about supporting people to consider what may be causing distress and to think creatively of ways to feel better. McEvoy, Eden and Plant (2014)[4] use the term 'empathic curiosity' to promote meaningful communication in the here and now with people living with dementia.

'Empathic curiosity' is a great term for a range of skills that include empathic listening; genuine interest; listening to verbal and non-verbal cues; being aware of metaphors; being calm; being fully present in the here and now; being self-aware and valuing the person and the relationship.

When people lose their short-term (or in some cases long-term) memory or become unable to find the right words they certainly do cause a lot of confusion amongst professional carers and families.

Much communication skills training in dementia care starts by focusing on reminiscence packages, which have their place. But individuals need different approaches. We need to listen more, with openness, to things we may never completely understand.

Defects, disorder, diseases…can play a paradoxical role, by bringing out latent powers, developments, evolutions, forms of life that might never be seen, or even be imaginable, in their absence… One may be horrified by the ravages of disease, one may see them as creative too – for if they destroy particular paths, particular ways of doing things, they may force the nervous system into making other paths and ways; force on it an unexpected growth and evolution. This other side of development or disease is something I see, potentially, in almost every patient.

(Sacks 1994)[5]

Confusion and searching may be opening minds. Did you remember that point?

Activities to support people who seem confused

These activities are simple and effective. They do not require much instruction, which makes them accessible and calming. They can be done individually, or in small groups as a social activity.

PATCHWORK PAINTING

Patchwork painting is a form of painting we developed to use with people diagnosed as living in mid to late stages of dementia. Whilst some people happily continue painting on blank canvas, others prefer to have guidance. Initially we tried using 'painting-by-numbers' sets, but these were unsatisfactory due to confusion over numbers.

People of all ages and all abilities enjoy patchwork painting. The readymade areas to be painted offer a level of comfort to people who do not feel confident about being faced with a blank canvas. We take a simple and recognisable shape (a cat, a bird, a chair) and turn it into a patchwork painting that is easy and satisfying to do.

You will need:

○ an image with a good outline

○ tracing paper

- ○ pencil
- ○ canvas board
- ○ acrylic paints
- ○ stiff bristle brushes
- ○ protective covers.

Trace the image onto tracing paper. Transfer the image to a canvas. You or your co-artist can now draw a few lines inside the shape to create 'patches'…and start painting different colours in the different patches.

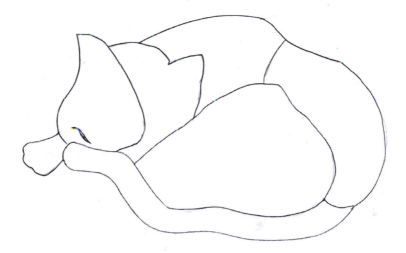

Figure 6.1: Patchwork cat

You could paint the background one solid colour, or you could divide that up into blocks of colour as well. The trick is to make sure that the colours you use for the main image are different from the background colours.

When the painting is dry, use a black or silver marker pen to outline the patches and main image. This really lifts the painting from the background.

WHICH PAINTS TO USE?

Although ordinary poster paints or waterbased paints wash out of clothes, we prefer to use acrylics. The colours are more stable and vibrant, and the paint dries more quickly. But they do stain clothing. Wear aprons and roll your sleeves up.

Acrylics dry fast, so only squeeze a little paint out of the tube at a time. You can put paint onto yogurt pot lids, or old china plates or a plastic palette.

Acrylic paint does not need water. You may want to use water to clean the brushes between colours, unless there is a likelihood of water being tipped over. If so, use separate brushes for separate colours, with a rag cloth to wipe the brushes if required. Use stiff bristle brushes. Floppy brushes are very frustrating with acrylics!

When acrylic dries it is permanent and the next layer will not mix with the dry layer in the way watercolour paints or pastels do. If you do want to blend colours, work fast before the colours dry. If you need to leave your paint on the palette, cover it with cling-film to stay wet for a day.

COLOUR MIXING

Sometimes it is better to discover colour mixes, but if someone wants to create a particular colour it is useful to know:

- red mixed with yellow = orange
- red mixed with blue = purple
- blue mixed with yellow = green
- blue, red and yellow = brown.

DÉCOUPAGE

We have found découpage is a natural progression from collage. Basic découpage is easy, looks good and does not require knowledge of art. The activity involves gluing gorgeous pieces of paper (colours, patterns, images) to decorate any object that appeals.

This is such a lovely activity to do with people at the table, or sitting in an armchair or in bed with a tray. The person is usually able to be involved at all stages of the activity. Another option is to do the activity in pairs. Given time to practice, we find participants become more able to do the task as the session unfolds. If at first a person seems uninterested, continue with your own découpage (not for the person, but for yourself). Being in the same space, showing how the activity is done, is a valid part of the process. Offer the activity again on another occasion, without pressure. It may be three or four times before the person feels able to give the activity a go and that is OK.

Whilst there are professional standards of découpage that require several layers of paper, varnish, sanding and more varnish, you can still create something stunningly beautiful with less effort. Show an example of a découpaged object (or an image). Choose the object you would like to cover, and place it on some newspaper or wipe-clean covering to protect the table and clothes.

Choose the patterned or coloured paper. If you choose a round or odd-shaped object to cover, it is better to use thinner papers and tissue paper that mould more easily.

Rip the paper into smaller pieces (rip, don't scissor cut, as the torn edges glue down much better). Magazine images can look good, as long as there is not a darker print on the other side that might come through when glued on.

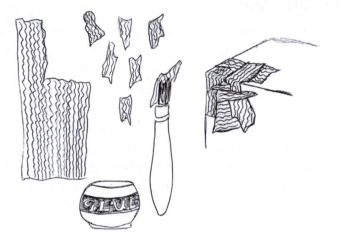

Figure 6.2: Découpage

Now get gluing! Brush glue onto a part of the object, then place a piece of paper over the glue. Glue again over the paper. The beauty of PVA glue is that it dries as though it is a varnish. It shines away and people sometimes mistake the découpaged objects for china or porcelain.

When the object is covered the way the person desires, check again for any gaps. There is satisfaction in discovering missed bits, and covering them over. Give the object a final coating of PVA glue and leave it to dry – or use a hairdryer if in a hurry.

An example of découpage teamwork: One man was content to rip paper, but less keen to do the gluing. His co-artist friend had painful arthritis, which prevented her from ripping paper. She was able to hold a glue brush and coat the object with glue. The man was happy to place the paper on the object, and so they were able to create the artwork together.

SIFTING AND SORTING

This is a more spontaneous activity that can help distract a person and create a calming environment. Sorting and sifting tasks can be found in folktales and myths where the heroine is given a seemingly impossible challenge, such as sorting poppy seeds from dirt, or wheat from barley.

In terms of metaphor these tasks are sometimes read as the ability to sort through emotions, or discern what matters. The tasks are always achieved. In the tale of Baba Yaga, a magic doll helps Vasalisa the Beautiful sort the poppy seeds. An army of ants helps Psyche sort the grain in Eros and Psyche.

Objects for sorting and sifting could include:

○ colourful plastic pegs, or plastic and wooden pegs

○ socks (into pairs)

○ beads (into sizes or colours)

○ paperwork (into page numbers, or paper size, or junk mail)

○ magazine pictures (into animals, people, or places).

Variations on this theme are folding laundry; sweeping; dusting; and sorting books on the shelf. Whether or not the tasks are achieved is not important. The activity is about comfort and feeling useful.

POETIC PHRASES

The words spoken by people with dementia are often poetic. Capture the amazing sentences and read them back to people. It is good to just savour the poetic nature of the words together.

○ 'My mind is like a sieve and I can see through the holes to the stars.'

○ 'You are on your knees for me. I bless you. Flower of the carpet.'

Some phrases are humorous and pertinent:

○ 'You dye your hair, but you do not change your waist. How so?'

Read poetry and prose that people may be familiar with, or by descriptions of experiences they can relate to:

These days I just can't seem to say what I mean [...]. I just can't. Every time I try to say something, it misses the point. Either that or I end up saying the opposite of what I mean. The more I try to get it right the more mixed up it gets. Sometimes I can't even remember what I was trying to say in the first place. It's like my body's split in two and one of me is chasing the other me around a big pillar. We're running circles around it. The other me has the right words, but I can never catch her.

(Murakami 2007, p.286)[6]

COLLAGE ON THE INSIDE

This is a variation on the collage in Chapter 1. Instead of having a blank page to fill, create a recognisable shape to be filled in with various materials. This could be the head of an animal or the shape of a vase, for example. The paper or material is glued inside the shape. If the person's artwork goes over the edge of the outline leave it all to dry, and when complete, the head or vase shape can be cut out of the paper and placed on a different colour background. These collages can be so effective, even using just two or three contrasting colours.

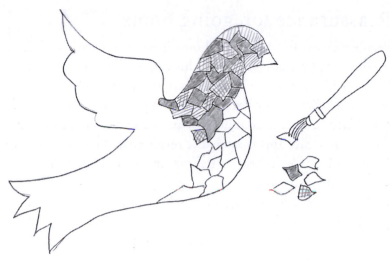

Figure 6.3: Collage of a bird

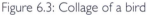

MATCHING SOUNDS WITH IMAGES

This is a sight and sound activity that requires preparation, but can be added to each week. This would work well on an iPad or a phone that can record sound and images.

1. Take photos and sound recordings of various implements or sounds in nature: kitchen appliances, walking on gravel, running water, the sea…
2. Print the photos (or use relevant magazine images). Spread the images out.
3. Play the sounds randomly.
4. Match the images to the sounds.

This can also be used as a basis for story-making, or creating poetry about the images and sounds.

Reassurance for 'going home'

People may ask to go home. If home is where they are, and there is no other physical place to go, this can become very upsetting. It is difficult for family carers (or care staff) when someone with dementia believes they are in the wrong place and that 'home' is somewhere else. It is common for people to tell the person that they *are* at home. This is rarely the response that the person with dementia is ready to hear or believe. In fact, it is more likely to cause further distress.

'Reassurance for going home' offers a range of strategies to help alleviate the distress. The main purpose of these responses is to soothe the person and find a way in which the person can connect in this moment.

Note: Carers and support staff sometimes confuse 'here and now' and 'this moment' with reality orientation; they think it is about getting the person to be in this present day, with all the facts about the date, and who the president is, or what the person had for dinner just now. It is not about that! Being in the here and now is about this breath, this connection, this sound, this feeling, this thought, this hand, this taste, this togetherness, this love, this peace... It is about beingness.

The validation approach to reassurance

Acknowledge that the person wants to go home. Resist all temptation to argue that they are home, or that they cannot go home. Tune in to the feeling of 'home'. Show that you understand what 'home' is. Ask the person more about home, for example: 'Home...that's the place where the heart is. Home is where the heart is. Home is the place where you feel safe and warm. Tell me more about home...'

Listen to what the person says, for they may offer you clues as to what their needs are, such as the need to feel protected or loved, which you can give; or the need to sort something important that you can help them list; or the need to see someone, when you can help them revel in all the things they love or like about that person; or the need to switch off the gas, which you can suddenly 'remember' you need to do yourself, and ask them to come and help you.

'Home' might have a spiritual meaning for the person: the place of ever-after. Sometimes in late stages of dementia people may act as though they are being 'called' by someone…perhaps hearing an old memory, or hearing thoughts about it being time to go home now. These are very delicate and sensitive times that require a lot of compassion and reassurance.

It may be appropriate to offer a prayer for home. This type of blessing helped one person feel more relaxed: 'Bless my home and keep it safe. Bless my home and fill it with love and peace. Bless my home and know that I am there.'

When people are in highly anxious states, sometimes the best approach is reassurance combined with distraction. Try a familiar song, or channel the energy of anxiety into a physical activity, such as preparing for the next meal. Sometimes going for a walk can help to alleviate the tension. One family carer talked about driving around with his relative who was searching for home. He occasionally stopped the car and wondered aloud if that was her home or not. As he neared their street he declared his surprise and relief that they had found her home. This ended with great pleasure and a cup of tea.

If nothing is really helping and you feel yourself becoming distressed, try using a chant or comforting sentence for yourself that is spoken quietly. You could use a chant as shown in Chapter 9 (see page 177) or a sing-song ditty made up on the spot that you repeat over and over: 'I am safe and so are you. We are finding our way through.'

A major factor in the escalation of anxiety or anger in someone with brain damage is their heightened sensitivity to other people's anxiety! So it is important for carers to know how to gain a state of calmness, which can help the other person feel better too. You can use chanting or self-talk that not only calms you down, but speaks also to the person who is distressed. Remember that the state of anxiety is highly uncomfortable, even painful, and the person will subconsciously be searching for a safe, calmer space…which might be you.

If you feel vulnerable to being hurt or to hurting, it is perfectly right to leave the room until the situation changes or you feel more supported. Do what feels right and keep listening to the person. It is OK if you need to call on a friend, a relative, or staff member for help.

Dementia teaches us the limits and expansions of ourselves as humans.

References

1. Kapura, M. and Bielaczyca, K. (2012) 'Designing for productive failure.' *Journal of the Learning Sciences 21*, 1, 45–83.
2. Normann, H.K., Asplund, K. and Norberg, A. (1998) 'Episodes of lucidity in people with severe dementia as narrated by formal carers.' *Journal of Advanced Nursing 28*, 6, 1295–1300.
3. Britton, B. (2014) 'Going places.' Available at http://d4dementia.blogspot.co.uk/2012/11/going-places.html. Accessed on 15 August 2015.
4. McEvoy, P., Eden, J. and Plant, R. (2014) 'Dementia communication using empathic curiosity.' *Nursing Times 110*, 24, 12–15. Available at www.nursingtimes.net/nursing-practice/clinical-zones/mental-health/dementia-communication-using-empathic-curiosity/5071690.article. Accessed on 15 August 2015.
5. Sacks, O. (1994) *An Anthropologist on Mars: Seven Paradoxical Tales.* Kindle edition (2011). London: Picador.
6. Murakumi, H. (2007) *Blind Willow, Sleeping Woman.* London: Vintage Books.

◦ 7 ◦

SUPPORT FOR MENTAL AND EMOTIONAL WELLBEING

Life feels good when we are tuned into feelings of resilience, hopefulness and wellbeing. People sometimes feel these emotions cannot exist after a diagnosis of dementia, but this is not the case. Feeling good is not tied up with what is going on…although we often think it is! Feeling good is far greater than any of the conditions we may be experiencing. How we get to that place is the subject of this chapter.

Imagine knowing that each day is a day to make the most of. What does that mean? What would make the most of your day?

- spending quality time with someone

- smelling the flowers

- noticing things that make you feel good

- being kind to yourself

- being kind to others

- noticing the sun rise or the sun set

- painting that picture

- making that meal.

Making the most of a day is never about our fears and anxieties, the worries and losses. But the negative feeling states occur when people focus their attention, understandably, on the things that make them feel low.

The following is a list of reasons that people living with dementia and their family members have given for why they feel depressed or fearful:

- I'm losing my life

- I'm losing my wife/husband/mother/father

- I'm scared of not being able to cope

- I don't want our days to end like this

- This isn't the retirement we had planned

- I don't want to be a burden to anyone

- I don't want to be burdened with all that responsibility

- I can no longer follow my dreams

- I don't want to end up in care

- I'm scared I won't recognise anyone

- I don't think I have the strength to look after him/her

- I feel cheated!

- I am angry that this has happened to me/us

- I'm scared I won't be able to communicate

- I don't want to be left behind

- I don't want to be left

- I feel powerless

- I can't see any reason to go on living

- I am scared that no one will see 'me' anymore

- I am afraid of being of no use to anyone anymore.

This is not a definitive list…because it is endless. When people feel these strong and difficult emotions there is a sense of being in a bottomless pit. People may experience deep sadness, even mourning, for all that could have been, and will not be. There may be profound anger about the unfairness and injustice of being 'chosen' by the illness or disease.

People may experience guilt about becoming ill: 'Maybe if I had done this instead of that; maybe if I had taken more exercise; eaten more blueberries; not taken on that contract; been more of something or less of something'. Sometimes the fear is about stigma – a deep sense of shame, or the fear of being treated only in terms of the dementia.

Family caregiving can also be very stressful. Family members sometimes speak about feeling trapped and tired. Trying to do the right thing for someone else is difficult when you are feeling so low and unsupported. On self-reported wellbeing scales, many course participants initially score low for feeling optimistic, relaxed, confident, or interested in new things. Studies show that caregiving can result in poorer health (Pinquart and Sorenson 2007;[1] Schulz and Martire 2004[2]).

Without mental and emotional wellbeing, people struggle. But things are changing; changes are occurring at global, national, community and personal levels as awareness grows and ideas arise – and we are all part of that process.

Dementia-friendly communities are developing all around the world. These are areas where people living with dementia feel included and supported to contribute to community life. This involves individuals, businesses, shops, banks, organisations, transport services and faith communities learning how to support people living with dementia.

In 2012, Britain's Prime Minister set a challenge to have 20 cities, towns and villages signed up to become dementia-friendly communities within 3 years. The response was huge. In 2015 there were over 82 areas signed up. The British Standards Institute developed a publicly available standard (PAS 1365:2015 Code of Practice for the Recognition of Dementia Friendly Communities in England, BSI June 2015)[3] that supports Alzheimer Society's recognition process of a dementia-friendly community.

Meanwhile, Alzheimer's Australia has developed a freely available dementia-friendly business toolkit and the dementia-friendly community toolkit, complete with action plan templates and helpful checklists.[4]

It is always good to begin by asking the people living with dementia and their families about their ideas for a dementia-friendly community. They know what feels supportive and what does not. The elements required for a dementia-friendly community might be physical, emotional and social. People need good lighting and clear signs as well as to be treated with kindness and patience.

Many UK high street stores, including Marks and Spencer, Argos and Homebase, are helping staff become more dementia aware. Some shops and banks offer a quiet area for people who need it, or check-outs with staff who can spend more time helping the person with their money or packing. These changes are happening all around the world.

Family carer programmes support relatives in learning how to care and support someone through changes to end-of-life care. See endnotes for further information. Family carers and care staff want to do their best and to feel more confident about caring, and more resilient about coping.

Staff learning programmes help people deliver person-centred care, with empathy and compassion. Staff are learning how to make connections under any and all circumstances and how to support people through a wide range of experiences and changes in needs.

Sometimes people living with dementia prefer to build a new relationship for support. Befriender schemes[5] help people in the community, offering much needed companionship by face-to-face contact or by phone or letter. The contact may involve a friendly chat, or focus on a particular goal such as going for a walk or writing a life story. Depression may be a response to dementia and there are befriending schemes for suicide prevention.[6] All of these schemes rely on carefully selected and trained volunteers, some of whom may be carers or people diagnosed with long-term conditions with the time and capacity to support others.

There are growing numbers of dementia champions, friends and organisations offering support and advice. Campaigning organisations raise awareness and support research to advance our understanding of how brains work, as well as developing and testing drug therapies.

Individuals – you, me, and all of us who believe that things can be different – are supporting changes for the better. We can improve our own mental and emotional wellbeing, even whilst living in conditions that are less than ideal. When we find ways to change the way we feel, we show others what can be done. There is nothing as empowering as knowing that feeling better is possible for yourself – and it is.

We have seen people move from feelings of great loss and fear to deepest peace and laughter whilst all the conditions remained the same. The people still had a diagnosis of dementia. The family carers still had the task of caring. But they found their ways through by changing how they felt.

It may take a lot of practice. The brain's neural networks have been sending messages that have been around for decades. It takes time to establish new pathways. Whether you are a family carer or staff member, or someone diagnosed with dementia, the following activities create tracks towards better feelings.

Creativity is a process of bringing something new into existence. Let's begin.

MAP OF THE HEART

People sometimes describe emotional wellbeing as feeling fulfilled, contented, confident or hopeful. Happiness and elation may also feature, and a sense of the heart singing. This beautiful activity is about creating a map of things that make your heart sing.

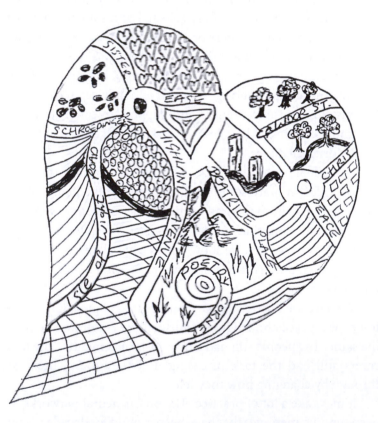

Figure 7.1: An example of a 'Map of the heart'

First list a few ideas under the following categories that you have experienced as positive or uplifting in your life, even if your heart currently feels heavy:

- Places that have given me joy
- People who have inspired me
- Objects I love or have loved
- Animals I love or have loved
- People I love or have loved
- Interests that have given me pleasure
- Ideas or beliefs that have sustained me.

Draw a heart shape on paper. The size depends on how much information you would like to add to it. Draw roads or tracks across the heart at various angles. Some roads may start or end outside the heart. Others are fully contained within the boundaries.

Before adding the written information, decorate the spaces between the roads. This could be done with paints or oil pastels, or using a felt pen to create different patterns within the spaces.

Decide where to place the names of people or places, etc., along the roads. If you have images of elements you listed, these could be glued onto the heart.

'Map of the Heart' is an activity that can be done before or after exploring poetry about the heart. People may be inspired by phrases or poetry to use different shapes for the heart map:

> My heart as a silver bowl with intricate patterns.
> My heart as a castle with high, turreted walls.
> It has a bronze covering inlaid with silver,
> originally gilt;
> the sides are decorated with openwork zoomorphic
> panels depicting events in the history
> of an unknown religion.
> The convoluted top-piece shows a high
> level of relief articulation,

as do the interworked spirals at the edges.

from 'My Heart' by Billy Collins (2001)[7]

GIFT MAKING

The giving and receiving of gifts is known in all cultures. People who are cared for may not have opportunities to give to others. This has been a strong feature in our work. We meet people who have a lot of love to give, but lack the means to express it.

It is more blessed to give than to receive.

(Acts 20:35)

When we are in a position to give to others, we are clearly privileged. Gift making can be done at any time and at any stage of dementia. It is useful to have a stock of wrapping paper (colourful or plain brown paper that can be decorated), with sticky tape, scissors, and ribbon or string.

Just wrapping things that are already in the house to give to family members can make a simple gift. A bar of soap, or a pretty napkin, or a pencil will do. The activity is really all about the process of wrapping. People in late stages of dementia rarely get the chance to wrap a present. People can usually hold the paper in place or wrap string around the paper. It is wonderful to create a sense of excitement about the surprise for a recipient.

A more involved gift is the making of a meaningful trinket box. This could be made from the treasure chest pattern in Chapter 1 (or use other small boxes to decorate). Discuss who the gift is for – a family member or friend or care staff. Cover the box in paper or paint, using colours or patterns that might suit the person receiving the gift. Line the inside of the box with more paper or material.

The gift inside the box could be any number of things chosen by the person. We create a lot of boxes about inner peace, so a feather or a pebble could work well. Sometimes the person is able to write.

A small booklet or letter inside the box is very special. Whatever the gift is, the recipient is likely to be genuinely touched. There is also pleasure in giving. Whether or not the activity is remembered is not important. What matters are the feelings during the process.

> It's not how much we give but how much love we put into giving.
>
> (Mother Teresa)

Mindfulness

Mindfulness is the quality of awareness that helps us calmly notice how we are responding or feeling in this moment of now. It is a state of acceptance of what 'is' in this instant, by just noticing it. Mindfulness practice allows people to gain some distance from the stress and anxiety they may be feeling about a situation. Rather than being caught in the escalation of anxiety or despair, it is possible, with practice, to become the observer of the situation.

By switching to the observer mode we give our minds a rest from habitual thoughts and reactions. We become fully consciously aware of our thoughts, feelings and bodily sensations without judging them as good or bad. This non-judgement reduces stress and anxiety, even though the situation remains the same.

> Mindfulness is about changing the way we relate to our experiences, not about changing those experiences.
>
> (Sinclair and Seydel 2013, p.62)[8]

The practice of mindfulness uses various tools such as meditation, mindful breathing and reflection. Relaxation is a welcome outcome as mindfulness techniques help the body and mind feel calmer.

Whitebird *et al.* (2012)[9] used a mindfulness-based stress reduction programme (MBSR) over an eight-week period with family carers. The study was done in comparison to a non-mindfulness intervention. Results showed that participants of the MBSR programme reported improvement in overall mental health, stress reduction and decreased depression, even though there were no changes in the caregiver situation. Mindfulness training has also been found to support people diagnosed with neurodegenerative disorders (Paller *et al.* 2014).[10]

The following is an example of a mindfulness meditation inspired by Thich Naht Hanh (2001, p.42).[11]

APPRECIATION OF AN APPLE

Feel the weight and shape of a fresh apple in your hand. Turn the apple in your hand. Feel the texture of its skin, the smoothness, the bumps and dents. As you hold the apple, notice your breathing.

> Rest your hand(s) holding the apple in your lap and breathe in slowly.

> Breathe out and allow your shoulders to relax a little.

> Breathe in, notice the weight of the apple in your hand on your lap.

> Breathe out, allow your shoulder muscles to relax a little more.

Hold the apple closer and notice the richness of skin colour. Consider the tree from where this apple came. Imagine the tree's growth through all the seasons year after year. See the tree in spring, summer, autumn and winter, and back to spring with its branches full of apple blossom. And from the flowers came the fruit. And from the fruit came this apple now in your hand.

Appreciate this opportunity to hold the apple in your hand. Notice your hand holding the apple in this moment. There is the apple and there is your hand holding the apple. Bring the apple to your mouth and take your time biting into the apple. Notice the sensations – the sound, the touch, the liquid and solid, the taste, the smell, your tongue, your teeth, your mouth. All these elements combine in the moment. Appreciate this opportunity to eat mindfully.

This same process can be used for any activity. It becomes an uplifting experience.

LETTERS TO THE DIS-EASE

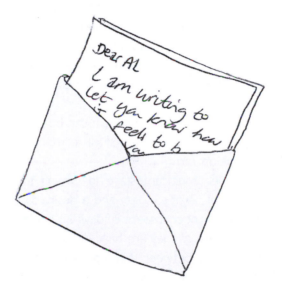

Figure 7.2: Letter to AI

Writing a letter to yourself can be very therapeutic. Many students have enjoyed writing letters from their imagined future 80-year-old selves, offering advice and guidance to the person they are now. Their words are insightful, tender and moving. Even though the letter writer and the letter receiver are the same person, there is a clear exchange that makes the letter receiver feel better. It is a way for the person to hear his or her innermost wise thoughts and to feel a sense of being on the right track.

Writing a letter to disease (or dis-ease) is a different form of therapeutic letter writing. The writer is usually the person affected (i.e. the person diagnosed with dementia), but can also be a family member. People can have scribes if the physical act of writing is not possible. The letter begins by expressing to the disease how it feels to be living with it. Some people give the disease a name to make it seem more like writing to a person. Once the person has vented all their feelings about the disease, they might want to end the letter there.

What to do with the finished letter is a personal choice. Sharing it with other people can help increase understanding of the experience and raise awareness about ways to support the person. Burning or shredding the letter can feel extremely cathartic. It can be empowering to purge oneself of all bitterness and anger towards the disease and have no trace of it left.

Keeping the letter is another option. It can be part of a personal record of change. Or perhaps the letter will form the basis of a story or other expressive art form.

There is another important stage in writing to the disease. This comes from a place of curiosity and a desire to build bridges. Some people find they need a space of days or weeks between the first and second letters, as they are highly contrasting experiences. There is a big difference between thinking about dementia from the perspective of anger and loss, and thinking about it with a sense of interest and hope.

The second letter asks the disease who it is, how it came here, or how it feels to be here, and what it wants? It is less judgmental than the first letter. The writer aims to be as open-minded as possible. He or she may start asking questions not thought of before, such as, 'Does my brain feel like a good place for you to be living in?' 'Is there something you want to tell me?'

It can be useful to think of the disease in terms of a young thing that gets up to tricks: 'I've noticed you like playing games. Where do you put all the words I can't find?' 'Is there a way we can share my brain nicely?'

The letters can be deeply poignant or outrageously funny... but the aim is to keep opening up to different perspectives and possibilities. Every new thought can lead to another. This process helps build new neural pathways, stimulating imagination and creativity – but more than that, it offers a greater sense of empowerment.

Is there a Stage 3 – does the disease write back to the person? This can only really work if the disease is seen as having a benevolent and kindly nature, which is not a common view. If the disease is seen only in terms of negativity, the letter from dementia may not be worth writing or receiving. If, however, the disease can be seen in terms of teaching us something, then the letter may contain exceptional words of wisdom.

APPRECIATIONS

List everything that you are grateful for and read it through to yourself or to the person you support. Share the joyfulness of all that is supporting you to live. Notice the things that continue with or without any effort from you. Gain a sense of being the recipient of many valuable experiences and things in life.

> I appreciate that the sun rises and sets every day.

> I appreciate hearing my favourite music every day.

> I thank the person who wrote that music.

> I appreciate the technology that helps me hear the music.

> I appreciate my home.

> I appreciate the things I have and the love I have.

> I appreciate all that is here and now.

Music

We know music reaches people. Creativity connects on an emotional level. Our brains process music across different areas (emotional, motor skills, visual, sound, language, and memory). If one part of the brain is damaged, another area may still be able to make a connection. We regularly meet people who have not spoken for a long time, but whose voices become loud and clear with a familiar song.

Stress is a barrier for positive communication, so anything that can reduce stress is important. Bradt and Dileo (2009)[12] explain that listening to music may reduce heart rate, high blood pressure and anxiety.

Way back in the 1950s Meyer (1956)[13] studied the emotional effects of music, showing that dopamine levels increased when people anticipated a particular part of the music they were listening to. Dopamine helps us gain a sense of reward and pleasure.

You may be familiar with that pleasurable anticipation for a familiar chorus, or when a piece of music feels as though it will take off. Examples include:

- Carl Orff: 'Carmina Burana – O Fortuna' (1936)

- The Ronettes: 'Be my baby' (1963)

- David Bowie: 'Life on Mars' (1971)

- Bon Jovi: 'Livin' on a prayer' (1987)

Keep adding tunes to your personal playlists in Chapter 3.

Feeling better can happen in a variety of ways, regardless of the situation you are in. This is easier to say when not in the depths of depression, but know that it is possible for you (or the person you care for) to find ways back to joyfulness. Creative activity, social networks, physical exercise, self-efficacy and compassion all help.

Endnotes

Courses by Creativity In Care, developed by the author, are taught through a creative process.

'Creativity in Dementia Care' is for staff, carers and artists to communicate more creatively and inclusively, increasing quality of life and supporting personal needs. Fun and practical talks and workshops.

'The ART of caring for self and others' is for family carers (attending with or without the person they support), brought in by community or adult services. Feedback shows increased confidence and capacity to support individual needs, and increased resilience for handling changes that occur through illness, through to end-of-life care. Eight- to ten-week creative and supportive programme.

'Co-Creating Care' is a consultancy programme for care facilities seeking a culture shift with all staff involved. The programme supports underpinning knowledge in a number of specified SVQ and NVQ health and social care (adult) courses levels 2 and 3. Spread over six months, this is a highly engaging, creative and supportive course for individual care facilities.

For more information contact info@creativityincare.org or visit www.creativityincare.org

Other information and courses

Check with your local Alzheimer organisations or care facilities for news on local courses. Meanwhile here are further contacts found by doing an online search:

UK

The Alzheimer Society delivers 'Carer Information and Support Programmes' for family members and friends around the UK.

www.alzheimers.org.uk/site/scripts/documents_info.php?
documentID=1710

The Contented Dementia Trust delivers courses for families and friends, and for health professionals (usually run in Oxfordshire).
www.contenteddementiatrust.org/courses

The Social Care Institute for Excellence developed a free open online course for everyone involved in dementia care.
www.scie.org.uk/dementia/open-dementia-e-learning-pro
gramme

Dementia Challengers website is full of information for family carers.
www.dementiachallengers.com

Australia

Check Alzheimer's Australia for family carer courses.
https://fightdementia.org.au/support-and-services/services-and-
programs-we-provide/family-carer-education

University of Tasmania 'Understanding Dementia' MOOC is a free nine week e-learning course.
www.utas.edu.au/wicking/wca/mooc

The RDNS (Royal District Nursing Service) offers a free e-learning course 'Getting to know me- a dementia training package'.
www.rdns.com.au/research/getting-to-know-me-a-dementia-
training-package

United States

Various free online workshops and other courses, with support groups run by Alzhemier's Association across America.
www.alz.org/care/alzheimers-dementia-care-training-certi
fication.asp#elearning

Crisis Prevention dementia care specialists offer person-centred training for care partners (staff).
www.crisisprevention.com/Specialties/Dementia-Care-Specialists/Our-Programs/Care-Partner-Training

References

1. Pinquart, M. and Sörensen, S. (2007) 'Correlates of physical health of informal caregivers: A meta-analysis.' *Journals of Gerontology. Series B, Psychological Sciences and Social Science 62*, 2, 126–137.
2. Schulz, R. and Martire, L.M. (2004). 'Family caregiving of persons with dementia: Prevalence, health effects, and support strategies.' *American Journal of Geriatric Psychiatry 12*, 240–249.
3. Dementia Friendly Community information. Available at www.alzheimers.org.uk/site/scripts/documents_info.php?documentID=2136. Accessed on 12 October 2015.
4. 'Alzheimer Australia's dementia friendly business and community toolkits.' Available at https://fightdementia.org.au/national/campaigns/dementia-friendly-communities/toolkits Accessed on 12 October 2015.
5. *Befriender Schemes (UK)*. Available at www.befriending.co.uk
6. *Worldwide Befrienders for the Prevention of Suicide*. Available at www.befrienders.org
7. Collins, B. (2001) *Sailing Alone Around the Room: New and Selected Poems*. New York: Random House Paperback.
8. Sinclair, M. and Seydel, J. (2013) *Mindfulness for Busy People: Turning Frantic and Frazzled into Calm and Composed*. Edinburgh: Pearson Education Ltd.
9. Whitebird, R.R., Kreitzer, M., Crain, L., Lewis, B.A., Hanson L.R. and Enstad, C.J. (2012) *Mindfulness-Based Stress Reduction for Family Caregivers: A Randomized Controlled Trial*. Oxford: Published by Oxford University Press on behalf of The Gerontological Society of America.
10. Paller, K.A., Creery, J.D., Florczak, S.M., Reber, P.J., Mesulam, M.-M., Weintraub, S. *et al.* (2015) 'Benefits of mindfulness training for patients with progressive cognitive decline and their caregivers.' *American Journal of Alzheimer's Disease and Other Dementias 30*, 257–267.
11. Thich Nhat Hanh (2001) *A Pebble for Your Pocket*. Berkeley, CA: Parallax Press.
12. Bradt, J. and Dileo, C. (2009) 'Music for stress and anxiety reduction in coronary heart disease patients.' Available at www.ncbi.nlm.nih.gov/pubmed/19370642. Accessed on 15 August 2015.
13. Meyer, L.B. (1956) *Emotion and Meaning in Music*. Chicago, IL: The University of Chicago Press.

∘ 8 ∘

SUPPORTING INDEPENDENCE

This entire book is about working in ways that honour individuals so that they can comfortably be who they are. This process requires movement between states of independence and interdependence, depending on circumstances and context. The activities in the book promote a sense of discovery or opening out from usual thoughts. Independence is about freedom.

People may be in the privileged position of being independent, but if their thoughts are focused on restrictions, limitations and negativity, their state of independence makes little difference to their quality of life. What helps us experience independence or support others in their independence?

- keeping our minds open to other perspectives

- thinking and responding creatively

- dwelling in the land of possibility

- never making assumptions about limitations.

Many people diagnosed with dementia continue to work, drive and live independently in the early stages of the disease, which can be for many years. Open and honest discussions early on (or even before diagnosis) can help families through the moral and ethical dilemmas that start to emerge if disease affects cognition and ability more significantly. (See page 173–174 regarding advance care plans.)

The notion of independence is highly valued in western culture. People want to be free from external control; free to be themselves under any and all circumstances. The freedom to think, feel, say and do what feels right for ourselves gives us a sense of inner integrity and confidence. Many people living with dementia are finding ways to be heard, and teaching others how to help them live more independently.

Independence is the opportunity and freedom to make choices about personal welfare. As world cultures create more dementia-friendly communities that give time (and timely support), people can successfully live independently, with and without family for many years. Two-thirds of people with dementia already do.

Factors that help to maintain independence

Being active and engaged with life. Learning new things keeps the brain active, as well as supporting emotional wellbeing. Learning can take place in formal settings, such as inspiring evening college classes or Internet-based programmes. Many courses offer options for studying without aiming for the qualification. Some offer certificates of attendance. Informal learning can happen anywhere, as shown in Chapter 4 in the section about bird-watching or stargazing. Learning can be as social or as private as you wish it to be.

Physical exercise is important. Not only does oxygen support brain function, but exercise will help us maintain strength and independence for longer.

Talking through strategies and plans with a trusted other. This is perhaps one of the most sensitive areas for people with a passion for being independent. It is a conversation that needs to start before illness makes the discussion difficult. Strategies are needed, for example, around electrical and fire safety; driving; becoming lost; or forgetting to eat.

In the UK the Driver and Vehicle Licensing Agency (DVLA) has a section on driving with dementia (or any organic brain syndrome). Decisions about driving rely on medical reports and are subject to annual review. Driving needs to stop if a person has poor short-term memory, disorientation or poor judgment of speed and distance.

The Fire Brigade/Department is able to assess homes and give advice on fire risk prevention. Fire safety staff are becoming more aware of risks posed by people who have cognitive difficulties or perception difficulties. Some people are advised to remove toasters at night, or disconnect the oven, but these are all individual and changing scenarios that need reviewing. Most advice is about ensuring that smoke alarms, heat detectors and carbon monoxide alarms are installed, and that fire exit routes are kept clear.

Technological assistance

We live in an age of technology that can support a range of situations. Satellite navigation systems help us to find our destination; recorded messages on timers remind people to take their medication; emergency buttons can call for assistance; clocks can tell whether it is morning or afternoon; doors can prompt you to 'remember your keys'; and automatic calendars always know what day it is.

Safety devices include pendant alarms and bracelet locators that alert someone if, for example, the person with dementia has gone beyond a specified radius. There are mats that alert carers if someone has got out of bed or stepped out of the front door, and devices that indicate if blood pressure or agitation level has risen.

We always need to consider ethics and consent issues before using interventions that reduce privacy. It is far better when interventions are in keeping with the person's wishes. The use of assistive technology needs to be regularly reviewed to assess problems and benefits.

The Dementia-Friendly Technology Charter is based on findings developed by Tunstall Healthcare with a large working group, published by the Alzheimer's Society (2014).[1] The charter aims to help every person with dementia have the opportunity to benefit from technology appropriate to his or her needs. It also outlines and promotes the implementation of high-level principles to help organisations provide best practice services to people with dementia.

Technology offers people a lot of enjoyment. Tablets and iPads are more popular now. People can see images, speak with family and watch home videos more easily.

Social life

Part of being independent is choosing who to spend time with and when. Some organisations offer dementia-friendly cafés to meet with other families or individuals living with dementia. There are many public groups and organisations that can be explored too: social art groups; nature walks; gardening groups; Men in Sheds; singing; religious groups, etc. There are often public talks and lectures in local libraries or colleges that may be of interest. Consider joining a board or committee of one of the organisations that offers services to people with dementia, or being a volunteer.

There are online forums (for example, on Twitter) that you can join for discussions and chats on any topic. (See 'Resources' at the end of this chapter.)

Living at home

If you live on your own and notice that sometimes you forget how to work something, write the instructions for yourself. Consider making signs to tell you what is inside the different cupboard doors, or invest in cupboard doors that are transparent. Place a sign on the door to say 'Keys and Phone'.

Have a note in your wallet or pocket that says who to call if you are concerned about becoming lost or disorientated.

If eyesight and visual perception become affected, the way your home is decorated can help. Have plain, warm-coloured flooring, as patterns can become confusing. (People sometimes see 'holes' or 'worms' in patterned carpets.) Ensure that the threshold strips blend in, since otherwise these can appear like steps or cracks to cross. Make sure the seats are easily visible against the carpet (colour contrast). Have good lighting to reduce shadows. Make things as obvious and easy to see as possible.

Interdependence

Another aspect of independence is acknowledging and planning for interdependence and dependence. Interdependence is mutual reliance of people or organisations upon each other. The health care and support facilities rely on people needing their services. On a personal level, interdependence is about building trusting relationships and sharing information with each other. Care services today are directed to work in partnership with families and people needing care to co-create best quality care. This transition from a system that previously had such a strong power imbalance is taking time to adjust.

Sabadosa and Batalden (2014)[2] show that improvements in care are possible when everyone involved (families, patients, service staff) cocreates and codelivers the best care. This requires changes in outlook and ownership of care, a readines to collaborate, and a stronger focus on being together on a learning journey.

There is no one set way to care for every person. It is a continuous process that improves when people listen and learn from one another. Medical or care staff can share their knowledge and practice by being more open and transparent. Families and individuals can offer their insights and understandings by engaging more fully. By focusing on solutions and improved care, each person involved supports the person being cared for, who also has his or her contributions to make to the process.

Future care planning and lasting power of attorney are part of this process (see Chapter 9).

Growing older

Young people are diagnosed with dementia, as well as older people. Regardless of dementia, there is a general view that growing old is about depreciation and decline. Cohen (2006)[3] presents a different view.

He promotes the idea of older people developing wisdom and maturity: people gain more flexible and insightful thinking styles that involve values and integrate emotions and reasoning (the heart and the head). His stages or 'potentials' for mature age describe more hopeful prospects of growing older, in four phases of older growth and development. Whilst neurological disease may interrupt some of these phases, the concept of continuing wisdom is important. Through the creative process we see much wisdom in people with dementia.

Cohen's stages 1 and 2 cover the ages between mid forties and early seventies, when people are motivated by a sense of mortality (or freedom) to fulfil their dreams. A combination of emotional and cognitive intelligence mixed with social and life experiences (and an ability to make sound judgments) creates the wisdom that we associate with mature people. People may go so far as to shake off old thinking patterns, and try something completely new.

The last two stages span the ages between late sixties and end of life. This is a time of reflecting on and evaluating life.

People may want to share their wisdom or find a way to state or affirm what they have come to know about life. There may be a desire to find resolutions to old conflicts, but mainly there is a search for meaning and a desire to live well until the end. People of this age have a great many stories to tell or ideas to express.

Cohen is clear that different people experience different phases, but the main point is that older age can be a time for new experiences, quests, creativity and growth. This can be true for anyone.

Activities to support independence

It is interesting that, when living with a diagnosis of illness, being independent depends, at least to some extent, on the attitudes and focus of everyone else. This works well when people embrace person-centred approaches that fully respect and focus on the individual's abilities. Person-centredness creates opportunity with positive expectation, rather than (unconsciously) setting someone up to fail by putting pressure on him or her to be the way they were, or the way everyone else thinks they should be.

> To know what you prefer instead of humbly saying Amen to what the world tells you, you ought to prefer, is to have kept your soul intact.
>
> (Robert Louis Stevenson)[4]

LIFE-STORY BOOK

The identity activities in Chapter 1 are also important for supporting independence, particularly the life-story book.

JOURNALING

Keep a journal of your daily experience. Notice what feels good to you. Notice what helps you feel empowered. You could keep a factual journal about places you have been. Which places felt friendly and comfortable? You could use words and/or sketch the things you have paid attention to today.

Keeping a journal can be useful as a reminder of recent events. It also can form the basis of an online blog.

ONLINE BLOGGING

People write about the things they love or know about. Some blogs have images with little writing, others write pages. You may have an interest that you could share online, or you may want to blog about your experience of dementia. Take a look at what other people are doing. Ask yourself:

○   What am I passionate about?

○   What do I know about?

○   Do I want to teach others? Or share experiences that help others?

There are guides to blogging, and most people use wordpress to begin with. You would need to think of a name for your blog (a domain name that becomes the web address), and you would need to pay to connect to the Internet, but these do not cost very much. Ask what other people use, or look up 'how to blog' on the Internet.

COMMUNICATION BOOK

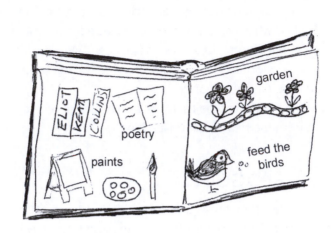

Figure 8.1: Communication book

Creating a communications book is an ongoing activity that will become more useful if cognition affects verbal communication. The communications book consists of words and clear images that show things that are important to you. Many people find these books useful to help communicate more clearly what they want. Think of it as a holiday phrasebook or pack of communication cards. It is perfectly natural to have back-up communication, and it reduces frustration.

You could make this as a physical booklet (or pack of cards) to have with you at all times; or create it as a digital book on a tablet. Think about your daily life and needs under various categories, and start taking photos or finding images that represent these elements. Cut or crop the main object out of the photos (or magazines) so that it is as clear to see as possible. (Too much background colour or paraphernalia will defeat the object of clear communication.)

Categories may include:

○   personal needs (toilet, bath, shave, hair wash, make-up)

- ○ food/eating (cutlery, plate, types of food)

- ○ clothing (underwear/tops/coat, etc.)

- ○ interests (books, paints, binoculars, pen and paper, crossword, music, etc.)

- ○ places (shops, library, home, bank, church)

- ○ travel (carpark, railway station, bus station, taxi).

Make it as comprehensive as you like!

SELF-PORTRAIT

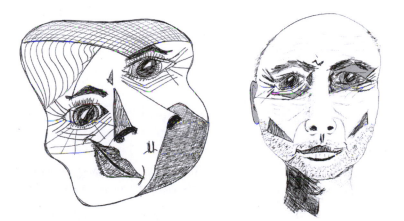

Figure 8.2 and 8.3: Self-portraits

Be an artist. You are an artist. Artists try things over and over again, perfecting their technique. Artists look at things in different ways. They play with colour and form. Self-portraits are absorbing and interesting. You could use any medium: charcoals, oil pastels or acrylic paints. You can create your portrait by drawing from a photograph, but it is often more fun and more effective to do it 'live'.

You will need a mirror in a place where you can see yourself well. Experiment with positions to be sure that you can maintain a steady position. You may want to do the self-portrait over a long period, or in several short sittings, so the position needs to be easy to hold.

Decide what facial expression you would like to paint, and whether you can create this expression every time you look at yourself. Initial paintings may be more about capturing the essence of you, so there is no need to get too concerned about these factors.

Draw or paint an outline of your head. Eyes are usually set about halfway down a face. Get the basics on the paper or canvas and fill in solid colours you can see, such as hair, skin, clothing. Experiment by choosing colours you like, rather than the colours you see. Where you can see shadows, use darker paint, and white or yellow for highlighting brightness. Step back from the portrait, or look at it in a mirror to get a fresh look as you work. Do as many self-portraits as you can.

The more you look at yourself, the more you will begin to see all the variations in colour and texture in your face, and the light and life in your eyes.

References

1. Alzheimer's Society (2014) *Dementia-friendly Technology Charter*. Available at www.alzheimers.org.uk/site/scripts/documents_info.php?documentID=2699. Accessed on 15 August 2015.
2. Sabadosa, K.A. and Batalden, P.B. (2014) 'Ten years of improvement innovation in cystic fibrosis care: The interdependent roles of patients, families and professionals in cystic fibrosis. A system for the coproduction of healthcare and its improvement.' *British Medical Journal Quality and Safety 23*, Suppl.1. i90-i94 doi:10.1136/bmjqs-2013-002782.
3. Cohen, G. (2006) *The Mature Mind: The Positive Power of the Aging Brain.* New York: Basic Books.
4. Stevenson, R.L. (1924) *An Inland Voyage and Travels with my Donkey in the Cevennes*. London: Heinemann, p.15.

Resources

DVLC guidance on driving

www.gov.uk/current-medical-guidelines-dvla-guidance-for-professionals-conditions-d-to-f#dementia-or-any-organic-brain-syndrome

Twitter forums

#AlzChat – every Monday at 8.00pm UK time/3.00pm Eastern Standard Time. This is a community of people who live with dementia, their relatives and interested staff. Hosted by Hilgos Foundation and Creativity in Care. Topics change every week.

#demphd – every Wednesday at 7.00pm UK time. Mostly dementia research students, but is open to all. Great topics.

SUPPORT FOR END-OF-LIFE CONNECTIONS

Caring for someone towards the end of his or her life is always a unique experience involving emotions that range from deep sadness to profound love. Preparation for death and dying may take many years, months or weeks. The experience is influenced by the nature of the disease; the environment and relationships; individual awareness, attitudes, beliefs, and 'readiness'.

End-of-life care supports people to live as fully as possible, adjusting to stages of illness and disease through palliative care. Care staff can help to relieve stress by being compassionate and respectful of individual fears and wishes and help people manage pain or discomfort. End-of-life care can be life-affirming, with a sense of appreciation for a life well lived.

There is a lot that can be done to prepare for death and dying. This may not make the situation any less painful or sad, but it can alleviate some of the stress faced by people who have not prepared.

- Celebrate life as often and as widely as possible.

- Seek reassurance about some of the fears people have about death and dying.

- Create an 'advance care plan' which describes preferences for how to be cared for in the event of being unable to communicate these desires.

- Establish a power/s of attorney for a) welfare and b) financial/property affairs in the event of incapacity.

- Create an advance directive (or 'living will') that defines the extent of medical intervention to be used, and any wishes around resuscitation.

- Sort insurances, wills, and other paperwork.

- Fulfil dreams and wishes.

- Leave a legacy or message for others.

It makes sense for all of us to have these preparations in place, even without a diagnosis of terminal illness. Most of these actions do not cost anything and can really help relatives if required in the event of an accident or illness. We hear too many stories of people feeling overwhelmed by the responsibility of trying to do the 'right thing' and wishing they knew what the person would have liked. Family carers generally do extremely well in supporting people, but having conversations earlier can be more beneficial.

The Lasting Power of Attorney (LPA) and Will documents do carry a charge. These seem to vary, so shop around. In the UK at the time of writing it costs £110 to register an LPA document. Some solicitors may offer a free will-writing service in exchange for a donation to a charity. However, there will be be solicitor fees involved in drawing up any documents, so ask for a quote. Things become a lot more expensive and difficult if the person does not have capacity to give consent, so do things before needed, or as early as possible. Note there are two separate LPAs to be registered (in England and Wales). One is for overseeing health and welfare, such as daily living, medical care or care home moves. The second LPA is for property and financial affairs, including bank accounts, bills, house sales and benefit collection.

In Scotland the registration is for a Welfare Power of Attorney (PoA), or a Continuing (financial) Power of Attorney, or a combination of the two.

If the person has lost capacity and there is no LPA or PoA in place, the Court of Protection becomes involved. Someone can then apply to be appointed a deputy to oversee the person's affairs, but this is more costly and there are ongoing fees to be paid to the Office of the Public Guardian. The Office of the Public Guardian can appoint someone who would not necessarily have been the choice of the family members.

The UK Mental Capacity Act 2005 assumes that every adult has mental capacity unless proved otherwise, and that each person has the right to make decisions. This includes the right to make decisions that may sound dangerous, such as parachute jumping, abseiling or jet-skiing!

Mental capacity is measured in terms of ability to understand and retain information, and to make choices based on that information. Some people with dementia may have mental capacity all their lives; for others the situation changes as the disease progresses. Many solicitors or lawyers understand the need to rephrase questions, use language that is clear, and communicate in a relaxed way, to give every opportunity for successful communication.

Power of attorney

In the UK this is called lasting power of attorney (England, Wales); enduring power of attorney (Northern Ireland) or continuing power of attorney (Scotland). These are legal documents that give authority for a named person or persons to act on behalf of another person in either specified matters or in all legal, financial and welfare matters.

Agreeing to power of attorney means having trust and faith in the friend or relative to always act well. This is by law what they must do. Any decisions taken on behalf of another person who does not have capacity, must be made in their best interests, and have the least restrictive impact on the person's freedom. Having a future care plan in place will be of huge help here.

Advance care plan

To start talking about future needs, you could begin by listing things you like now: favourite music, books and films. Then discuss which of these you (or the person you support) would always want to have available. The plan can be added to for other areas of care. It ensures that those around you know your hopes, even if you are unable to say what they are. The advance care plan is very personal, so it is unlikely to look exactly the same as anyone else's plan.

Things that need to be in your plan:

- name

- address

- date of birth

- your GP's name and contact details

- your signature (and witness to your signature)

- date of writing the plan (and any updates, dated)

- name and contact of any healthcare person or family member involved in discussions about these plans (if applicable)

- name and contact of next of kin or of person who has power of attorney for welfare or finance.

The rest of the plan is about your wishes and hopes for how you would be cared for if that was ever needed. See Appendix 1 for guiding questions. This plan is all about things that are important to you, the things you like or love, and things that relax you or make you feel good.

Have fun with your plan. Create a scrapbook or journal so that you can add ideas and stick in images of favourite things. The advance care plan is a 'living document', which means it grows and changes with you. Every New Year is a good time to check the plan, as most of us are thinking about what we want around that time.

Advance directives

An advance directive ('living will') makes clear an individual's wishes regarding resuscitation and medical interventions. The directive may be as simple as the following statement:

> If I only have a few weeks to live and am unable to communicate and have irreversible brain damage, or am in a coma, and unlikely to regain consciousness, then the treatment I want is for relieving pain and not treatment to prolong dying.

Once you start realising all the possibilities, the decision may not be so simple. People's lives can be prolonged, and in some situations that has enabled them to achieve something important, such as a connection to a lost family member. Life-and-death decisions need consideration.

Death and dying

Although dementia is regarded as a terminal illness, the prognosis is variable. Each person's experience of dementia depends on their previous mental and physical health, their current lifestyle and diet, and the nature of the disease. Death from heart disease, pulmonary disease, diabetes, or pneumonia due to a weakened immune system, is more likely to be on a death certificate than dementia, which means many people die with dementia, rather than of it.

Studies noted in a report by the European World Health Organisation show that 75 per cent of the general population would prefer to die at home (Davies and Higginson 2004, pp.16–17)[1] The Office for National Statistics (2011) shows that only 21 per cent of people die at home in the UK; compare with a similar figure for the USA (between 18 and 32 per cent).

Most people die in nursing homes or hospital. Whilst palliative care is improving in care facilities, it is clear that many people do not get the ending they would like to have. This may, in part, be due to family members feeling unable to cope with the death and dying of a loved one. It may also be that death and dying are regarded as a medical issue more than a social experience.

It is interesting (in western culture) that people do not spend much time with people who are dying. Perhaps this is about fear or a sense of being inadequate and just not knowing what to do or say. Some people say they are not at all spiritual so can be of no use to the person who is dying, and yet they attend the person's funeral. In *The Tibetan Book of Living and Dying*, Sogyal Rinpoche (1992)[2] talks about the all-important 'quality of presence' when carers are with people at their most vulnerable and extreme moment. This quality is being in the moment with the person, with an openness and ability to listen. This presence can be practised through mindfulness and breathing techniques.

Gentle physical care

Offering physical comfort can be soothing, such as gently brushing or combing hair, or offering a tender head massage. Holding hands and breathing together are calming ways to be together. (See also the activities in Chapter 3.)

Mouth hygiene is also important. The heart and mouth are directly linked. Poor mouth hygiene is associated with cardiovascular disease (*British Medical Journal* 2010)[3] and other systemic illnesses, such as diabetes, stroke, hypertension, myocardial infarction and aspiration pneumonia (Stein and Henry 2009).[4] If toothbrushing is too difficult or painful, the suggestion is to use a foam stick soaked in alcohol-free mouth rinse. Sipping water also helps keep the mouth clean.

Relatives (and care staff) may respond to death and dying with a range of feelings. Some people feel better able to cope than others. Kübler-Ross (1969)[5] highlighted five stages of grief that people may experience, from denial to anger, bargaining to depression, and finally acceptance. This can be a long process. Not everyone feels all these emotions, but it is important to allow yourself and the feelings of others to be heard with compassion.

People may like to see a spiritual or religious practitioner even if they did not previously think they would want to. Do your best to follow the person's wishes. Sometimes people fall asleep and move into death without speaking. Other people (who may or may not be religious) become anxious and ask if they will be forgiven. Sogyal Rinpoche suggests saying something reassuring and soothing like 'Forgiveness is already there. Can you forgive yourself now?' Having used this phrase with people who were worried before death, I have seen that the need for reassurance can be fulfilled and that death can be peaceful. Forgiveness of self can be an important part of dying.

Activities for end-of-life care

NATURE'S MUSIC

Some of the most relaxing and enjoyable sounds are found in nature. We sometimes take a handheld recording device out on walks to record birdsong, waterfalls, footsteps through leaves, or waves lapping over the pebbles. Soundscapes stimulate our imaginations. We watch people close their eyes and listen intently to the sounds, with smiles, or eye twitches, hands on heart, as their breathing becomes deeper.

You can find free online sites to hear a range of sounds such as frogs, birds, oceans, rain, cat purrs. There are also albums of natural sounds (forests, oceans, country gardens), and DVDs containing beautiful film footage of (for example) butterflies, swans and flowers, set to gentle music.

COMFORT CHANTS

Chanting is used all around the world. The repetitive nature of the sounds or words can calm agitated minds and help people feel more reassured.

Chanting may be done for spiritual practice, to feel more aligned with higher consciousness. The words can be prayerlike, or devotions to God. Other chants do not need to be religious, but can offer words of comfort and hope. They often use simple tunes. Speak the words first, and allow them to create a rhythm that becomes a tune – for example, 'Love is in my heart and comforts me.'

We find chanting slows the breath and reduces anxiety and fear. Some people use chanting to focus them in this moment, here and now. Paradoxically, the deepening relaxation can make people feel 'somewhere else'. The rhythmic repetition of sounds and words helps people move away from thoughts that are stressful.

You can make up chants at any time. Just say whatever words feel right – or use sounds rather than words. When one lady was crying and no one knew why, we began a slow and gentle chant, which she joined in with after a couple of minutes:

'On a day like today, may peace be in my heart.

Mmm, ahhh, mmm, may peace be in my heart.'

The word 'my' is used instead of 'your' simply so that the person does not need to change any words for the chant to be theirs. This is a personal choice, and you may prefer to use different words.

GENTLE PUPPETRY

Dying does not have to be quiet and serious all the time. Some people really enjoy a lively and colourful event at their deathbed. Children and animals can be great tonics, but are not always readily available. Puppetry is! Puppetry was originally for adults; for passing on religious, social and political news from village to village. Puppets are great for silent, emotional expression, for they are both poignant and humorous.

People may become more physically sensitive towards the end of life. Touch needs to be gentle, materials softer. We sometimes use soft animal puppets, or pieces of cloth knotted to create a head. The puppets can be animated around the person…drawing the person into another world. Watching a puppet explore the bed or items in the room engages us in the curiosity and wonder of everything.

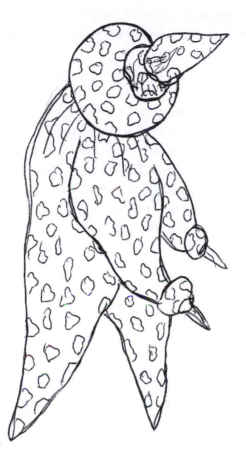

Figure 9.1: Scarf puppet

If short of materials, use a bed sheet or scarf to create a puppet. Hold enough of the middle of the material to tie it into a knot to create the head. Leave the end of the knot poking through to be the nose.

The rest of the material should contain four corners. One corner will fall in front of the head, one behind, one to the left, and one to the right. Take the left and right corners and tie each one separately into a knot to create hands.

Hold the puppet from behind the neck (below the centre knot) and allow the puppet to 'see' by tilting its nose in the direction of objects.

Use your other hand to manipulate one of the puppet hands to point to objects.

We become oblivious to regular objects. The puppet can highlight things in ways that renew our perspective. It is a playfulness that takes practice, because the puppeteer is breathing life into something. This requires being fully mindful of the puppet. For some people puppetry will be a natural ability.

Sometimes the person indicates a desire to be the puppeteer. Have two or more puppets available. Use puppets that can be washed (most soft puppets can be washed inside a pillowcase). Towards the end of life, it may be easier for people to let go of being self-conscious. There is often a 'playfulness' that is ready and willing to awaken.

LETTERS TO LOVED ONES

This is an activity that means so much to family carers and to staff in receipt of the letters. Even when the letters are very short, they represent a whole life.

Begin by talking about words of wisdom or thoughts that the person would like to pass to the next generation. Create a list of close family members or carers, gather envelopes and address them. You could make a card together, buy a card or use proper writing paper.

Some people are happy to write a note. It might be a family saying, some advice for living well, or a happy memory of someone. Sometimes people want to pass on a recipe or suggest a business idea. These messages may be as random as the person proposes.

If the person is too frail to write, he or she can dictate the note. But sometimes speaking and writing are not possible. Show the person the envelope and paper or card. They may indicate recognition of the activity. If this is the case, speak with the person about the idea of sending a card just to say 'hello' or 'thank you' or 'thinking of you'.

The person can be involved in choosing the card, maybe printing an image using a rubber stamp and printing ink, or marking the card with a heart or kiss.

SPACE TRAVELLER

Fairytales often end with the phrase 'happy ever after'. It can be difficult to imagine eternal happiness…but for some people that could describe heaven.

Trying to describe or explain foreverness is like trying to understand the billions and trillions of connections in our brains. The wonder of it all is enthralling. The infinity of space beyond our galaxy is beyond our comprehension. The knowledge that our brains contain numerous sensitive astrocytes – star-shaped neurons (Lee *et al.* 2014)[6] is astounding.

We can envisage the awe experienced by astronauts who get to see Earth from afar. They see the beauty and fragility of our world.

Being a 'space traveller' helps us realise things we cannot always appreciate here on earth. This activity is about imagining we are travellers of the universe, who can see Earth and other planets. We might want to express the 'happy ever after' or the beauty of stars and planets.

This can be done as a collage (see Chapter 1, p.20). Have a wide variety of magazines available for images (*Homes and Gardens*; nature; wildlife; space; travel; astronomy; *National Geographic*).

You may prefer to decorate large polystyrene balls with PVA glue and coloured tissue papers, making unique planets to hang from the ceiling. Before decorating a ball, thread wire though it (fold up the end with pliers to keep it in place). Make the other end into a hoop for hanging. Begin by showing images of astronauts and of the moon, the stars, the Earth and other planets.

When complete, ensure that the person can see the work from their bed. Hang planets from the ceiling, or pin the collage up there. Honour the thoughts and process that have gone into this creation.

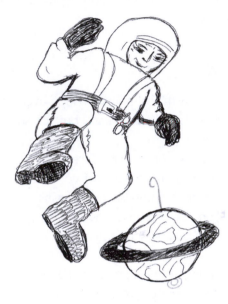

Figure 9.2: Planet balls

When working with people who are dying, we are working with people who know the essence of humanity.

The essence of humanity is love.

References

1. Davies, E. and Higginson, I.J. (eds) (2004) *The Solid Facts: Palliative Care.* World Health Organization: Europe. Available at www.euro.who.int/__ data/assets/pdf_file/0003/98418/E82931.pdf. Accessed on 15 August 2015.
2. Rinpoche, S. (1992) *The Tibetan Book of Living and Dying.* London: Random House.
3. de Olivera, C., Watt, R. and Hammer, M. (2010) 'Toothbrushing, inflammation, and risk of cardiovascular disease: results from Scottish Health Survey.' *British Medical Journal 340,* c2451.

4. Stein, P.S. and Henry, R.G. (2009) 'Poor oral hygiene in long-term care: Nurses must provide better oral care to older adults and patients with severe disabilities.' *American Journal of Nursing 109*, 44–51.

5. Kübler-Ross, E. (1969) *On Death and Dying.* London: MacMillan, pp.45–60.

6. Lee, H.S., Ghetti, A., Pinto-Duarte, A., Wang, X., Dziewczapolski, G., Galimi, F. *et al.* (2014) 'Astrocytes contribute to gamma oscillations and recognition memory.' *Proceedings of the National Academy of Sciences of the United States of America 111*, 32, E3343–E3352. doi:10.1073/pnas.1410893111. Available at www.ncbi.nlm.nih.gov/pmc/articles/PMC 4136580. Accessed on 15 August 2015.

° 10 °

SESSION PLANNING

Plans are ongoing and useful resources that help clarify what is important. They vary from a simple weekly meal plan to a complex five-year life plan. Developing a plan helps us to set our intentions. We can identify what we want to happen (our desirable expectations) and list ways to achieve those goals. The plan can be a motivational tool. It also gives us a record to measure progress by.

Life coaches use planning tools with their clients. These may focus on one particular area of life that the person feels is out of balance or the cause of unhappiness. Common areas are stress management and work/life balance. There are coaches and planners for fitness and wellbeing, business, retirement, personal image, and career changes.

Care facilities are used to creating short-term and long-term plans that cover various aspects of people's lives. Families or individuals who receive community support may also be familiar with the concept.

Most care plans focus on:

- physical and biological needs

- social and interpersonal needs

- emotional and mental health needs

- intellectual or interest needs

- spiritual or symbolic needs.

The overall aim is to ensure that the care is relevant to the individual's needs, person-centred and effective. The advance life plans (see Chapter 9) serve a similar purpose for end-of-life care and support.

The relationship with a care planner or life coach planner is one of trust. There are likely to be several care staff involved in a care plan. The person and/or their family need to feel comfortable about sharing information so their needs can be understood and responded to. All care staff and volunteers should be made aware of their obligation to maintain confidentiality of personal information.

This section is about planning for activities, but you could use it for other topics. It is always important to share the creation of the plan with the person being supported, without exception. They can indicate or say what they want. Even if verbal or sign language is not being used, the person has a right to be part of the process and may still understand what is being said. Even if they do not understand what is being said, the person may still be sensitive to the fact that you are including them, which helps build trust. Trust is essential for effective care.

Many staff and family carers now recognise the importance of offering activities and social events. To be effective and beneficial, the activities need to be relevant and meaningful to the individual/s. If a care setting puts up a timetable of weekly activities, this can look magnificent, but it needs to be of interest and benefit to the people in the care setting.

Many care settings offer activities that are well intentioned, but which are limited by the awareness or experience of the person leading the session. This can lead to an unintentional decrease in the participant's self-esteem. One example of this could be the painting of hands to cut out and glue onto paper to create patterns or shapes: the activity can be fun and it is certainly accessible, but if people feel embarrassed or diminished by an activity that they associate with nursery school, it is not an effective engagement.

If people want to create and paint shapes to glue onto paper, refer to the artist Matisse (pp.117–118). Look at his work. His methods are extremely accessible and highly relevant.

Planning for activities

Consider who the participants are and what their needs are. Focus on desirable benefits as identified by participant/s or carer/s – for example:

- increased sense of identity or self-expression

- enhanced social relationships and communication

- increased self-esteem

- improved mental stimulation

- maintenance of physical health

- increased relaxation, reduced anxiety.

Choose activities from this book to support those benefits, or design your own activities:

- increased sense of identity or self-expression – Chapters 1, 2, 5

- enhanced social relationships – Chapter 3. (Every chapter contains shared activities and activities to support better communication)

- increased self-esteem – Chapter 7

- improved mental stimulation – every chapter contains activities that stimulate the brain

- maintain physical health – Chapter 4

- increased relaxation – Chapters 6 and 9.

See Appendix 2 for a blank Activities Plan.

Reflecting on practice

The reflective journal is a space for you to think about the work and how you feel about particular aspects of the work. This helps build confidence and recognition of personal strengths. It is a private and personal document, it is also a place to let off steam.

The journal can be a notebook of thoughts, ideas, or sketches about your experience of the work. It does not have to be in writing.

It can be a structured activity, such as answering a set of questions (shown below), or it can be a way of conveying an overall sense of the work using imagery, colours and/or a sketch.

Either way, it is good practice to record your thinking as soon as possible after the work, and to date the journal entry. This helps to get a sense of how things are progressing or changing for you, as you look back over the journal.

Being aware of how *we* feel helps us be more aware of how others may be experiencing the projects we deliver. This in turn helps us see how to make improvements.

Guiding questions (just choose ones that seem relevant to you):

1. What did I enjoy about today?

2. What did I do well today?

3. What, if anything, did I feel didn't go so well?

4. What would I say about that from my inner wisdom self?

5. What would I like to do differently next time?

6. Was there anyone I felt irritated by? (Do not name the person.)

7. Can I let go of that and find a redeeming feature to focus on next time I meet them?

8. Was there anyone I felt I would want support with next time? (Do not name the person.)

9. What did I learn today?

10. What ideas would I like to try out?

Managing risk

Everything has some element of risk attached to it, including being sedentary. Creative activities may contain potential risks, such as ingesting materials, cutting fingers and staining clothes, so it is important to consider ways of managing the risks. These can be quite simple measures. Do a risk assessment for each activity (see Appendix 3).

If buying art materials from a store, ask if there are any warnings to be aware of. Some suppliers of paints and glues offer hazards information, so check online as well. The most common hazards (things that have potential to cause harm) in the activities in this book are scissors, glue and paint. The risks (the likelihood that they may cause harm) are variable, depending on the type of material, who is using it, and in what sort of environment.

It can be more fun and more useful to do a risk assessment with everyone involved in the activity. This ensures that everyone is aware, and creates a sense of self-responsibility. Sometimes people will suggest hazards that the facilitator had not thought of.

Equally, people can suggest ways of managing risks that enhance the safety of the activity.

There are always ways to manage the risks, such as using different materials (non-toxic/water-based); supervising the person; wearing protective clothing; having regular breaks.

Risk is an intrinsic element of being creative. Creativity is the process of making something that was not there before. Some artists create art that risks challenging society. Mostly they challenge themselves.

Living with dementia is also a risky business. You never know what to expect or how you will deal with it. There will be times when carers fail to support, and times when behaviour or speech by the person with dementia causes other people a lot of distress – but these are all useful learning points that can be managed better next time.

Dementia challenges us to see the world and ourselves differently. Creativity is an important part of learning how to live with what this brings. It strengthens communication and understanding. It helps us all to connect.

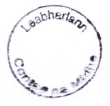

APPENDIX I
ADVANCE CARE PLANNING

The following questions are to help you create an advance care plan to ensure that those around you understand how you would like to be cared for if you were unable to explain. The plan can grow and change as your preferences change. The plan needs to have your name, address, date of birth, a witnessed signature and date of plan. It may also contain the name of your GP and any medical advisor involved. The plan is not a legal document, but it provides strong evidence of your wishes.

What makes me feel good… emotionally and socially?

- What sort of things, sights or sounds make me feel happy?
- Who is important to me… whether or not they are physically alive?
- What kind of music do I like? [Create a personal playlist.]
- What words do I like to hear? [Poetry, song lyrics, storybooks…]
- What are my favourite animals? What pets do I have? How do I want my pets to be cared for?
- The sort of landscape or nature places I love are…
- My favourite films are…
- What pictures would I like to have in my room?
- If I have moments of feeling deep sadness or become upset, I would like to have time alone to have a good cry *or* have someone hold my hand and comfort me…*or*…
- What sort of activities do I like?
- What kinds of activities do not interest me? (But I could still be invited to, just in case.)
- Do I like time alone, or do I prefer to be among other people?
- What sort of groups do I like?
- Do I like quietness or hustle and bustle?

What do I prefer physically?

- Double bed or single bed? What type of sheets or bedding do I like?
- How early do I like to rise?
- Bath or shower? Favourite toiletries?
- How long do I usually prefer to spend on the toilet?
- What are my favourite clothes? Colours? Styles?
- How do I like my hair to be?
- What is non-negotiable?
- How often do I like to eat? What are my favourite foods?
- What sort of breakfast do I like to have? What foods do I not want at all? Any allergies?
- What are my favourite drinks?
- Do I have any regular routine at the moment? [Describe it…]
- Where would I most like to live and be cared for? What's my second choice?

What spiritual needs do I have?

- What religious beliefs or comforting beliefs do I have?
- What brings me deepest comfort and peace of heart and mind?
- What do I want to help me maintain my spiritual wellbeing?
- What are my favourite religious texts or music or hymns?
- Are there any objects or icons that I like to have?
- What sort of funeral service would I like? Burial or cremation?
- Is there anyone I would like to speak with or connect with before I die?
- What words of wisdom or comfort would I like to leave for others?

APPENDIX 2
ACTIVITIES PLAN

Date of plan:	
Lead facilitator:	
Date of planned for activity:	
Time available:	
Name(s) of participant(s) and/or co-artist(s):	
Individual and/or shared work:	
Desirable benefits to focus on as identified by participant(s) or carer(s):	
Name of activity to support the benefit:	
Materials required:	
Identified hazards: (See risk assessment)	
Observation and feedback from session:	
Notes for future activity:	

APPENDIX 3

RISK ASSESSMENT FORM

Description of activity being assessed:	Name of assessor:
Location where activity will take place:	Name of company:
	Date completed: Date .... Signed .... Date .... Signed .... Date .... Signed .... Date .... Signed ....

STEP 1	STEP 2	STEP 3	STEP 4			STEP 5
List potential hazards here.	List groups of people who are at risk from the hazards you have identified.	List existing controls.	Calculate the residual risk, taking the presence and effectiveness of control measures into account.*			List further control measures necessary to reduce risk to an acceptable level.
			Severity (1 to 3)	Likelihood (1 to 3)	Risk rating	

* Risk rating = severity x likelihood

Note: Risk ratings of 4 or more are significant and require action.

INDEX

Page numbers in *italics* refer to figures.